# WOMEN's HEALTH IN GOA

## About the Editor

**Shaila Desouza** by professional training is a Fine Artist and Social Worker. She has been involved since 1987 in researching women's health. She has been involved with projects of the Ministry of Health and Family Welfare. She is currently at the Centre for Women's Studies of the Goa University where she is engaged in research, teaching, documentation and activism on issues related to women and children. She has been adviser to several government, semi-government as well as Non-Government Organisations in Goa and has to her credit several national and international publications.

# Women's Health in Goa

## A Holistic Approach

*Edited by*

**Shaila Desouza**

CONCEPT PUBLISHING COMPANY, NEW DELHI-110059

**Cataloging in Publication Data—DK**
*Courtesy:* D.K. Agencies (P) Ltd. <docinfo@dkagencies.com>

**Women's health in Goa :** a holistic approach
/ edited by Shaila Desouza.
p. cm.
Papers presented at a workshop held at Goa University in November 2002.
Includes bibliographical references.
ISBN 8180692566

1. Women—Health and hygiene—India—Goa—Congresses.
2. Women—Mental health—India—Goa—Congresses.
I. Desouza, Shaila.

DDC 362.108 209 547 99 21



ISBN 81-8069-256-6

First Published 2006



*Published and Printed by*
Ashok Kumar Mittal
**Concept Publishing Company**
A/15-16, Commercial Block, Mohan Garden,
New Delhi-110 059 (India)

*Phones* : 25351460, 25351794
*Fax* : 091-11-25357103
*Email* : publishing@conceptpub.com

# CONTENTS

## Sex, Sexuality and Reproductive Health



## Health and Human Rights Issues



## Neglected Today: Forgotten Tomorrow



## Novel Perspectives of Old Health Systems

# INTRODUCTION

*Shaila Desouza*

In November 2002, the Centre for Women's Studies, Goa University and the Goa State Commission for Women collaborated on a project titled Reaching Beyond Figures: State of Women's Health in Goa. Both the organisers opined that 'health' was not only a personal issue but, an economic, social as well as political one. Therefore, the first part of the project was a workshop, which invited wide-ranging perspectives on various themes concerning women's health. Participants at this event included doctors and other health professionals, lawyers, academicians, NGO representatives, government officials, activists, etc. For the very first time in Goa, the subject of women's health was being approached from some of these different dimensions. The workshop sought to look in particular at the impact of gender discrimination and poverty on health from childhood to old age and the impact of policies in a globalising world.

Goa's 'health statistics' and 'development' indicators have been considered one of the best in the country. And yet, these indicators do not reveal various areas of concern for the women in the State. The workshop therefore aimed to investigate women's health and interrogate what the existing statistics did not tell and present a more holistic picture. This publication is the final part of the current project, to make available to a larger audience the discussions that contributors to this volume have highlighted. This volume however is the beginning of another phase of work to be undertaken by the

Centre for Women's Studies, Goa University and the Goa State Commission for Women to improve the state of women's health in Goa. This volume in that respect is just the beginning.

The participation was very encouraging for both the days of the workshop and this volume is testimony to the quality of the presentations made. Despite busy schedules, the authors have made this volume possible.

The heterogeneity of the author's professional background has added to the diversity of approaches tied by the common concern for women's well-being. Some of the papers presented here do not focus on Goa but their inclusion has been felt necessary to throw light on often ignored issues.

The papers are grouped under six broad sub-heads

1. Overview of Health, Policy and Programme.
2. Mental Health Issues.
3. Sex, Sexuality and Reproductive Health.
4. Health and Human Rights.
5. Vulnerable Groups-Neglected Today, Forgotten Tomorrow?
6. Novel Perspectives of Old Health Systems.

Imrana Qadeer seeks to understand why motherhood in India even today remains unsafe. The issue of access and quality of health services needs to be linked to factors that lie outside the medical domain. Differentials across gender, class and caste need to be placed in the context of economic and social processes such as, a dwindling public distribution system, the move from food crops to cash crops etc. An understanding of women's health needs to combine medical scholarship with social sciences approaches to health. She makes a case for changes at the level of macro planning to improve women's health.

Pradeep Padwal in his contribution gives a detailed account of the different programmes that the public health system in Goa offers as part of the Reproductive and Child Health Programme.

The changing political set up in the last decade needs a critical view and Shalla Desouza's paper attempts a critique of the State Health Programme for women. She argues that decentralised participatory planning must reflect in the provision of 'quality services' and a definite change in the aggressive control of women's fertility through contraceptive device.

A neglected area in the mainstream literature on women's health is the issue of mental health. Four contributions in this volume redress that and remind us that many 'illnesses' of the body are intrinsically linked to the 'mind'. Prabha Chandra looks the needs of mentally ill women and proposes methods of better health care delivery that will deal with their unmet needs.

Vikram Patel's paper is based on a micro-level study in Goa. He finds that more than a third of women suffered from depression and anxiety disorders. Some reproductive somatic symptoms such as venereal disease (VD), like many other somatic idioms, could be associated with psychological morbidity (such as depression) and social problems. He draws attention to the enormous financial and social cost if these links are overlooked.

While most global efforts focus on improving maternal and child physical health, there has been a global disregard for the psychological well-being of the mother-infant dyad. Nandita de Souza, and Marcus Hughes argue that maternal mental health problems can seriously disrupt child development leading to enduring disadvantage in learning and socialisation.

Family violence could be another source of mental disorder and it impacts on the health of women and the community at large. Fiona Dias Saxena argues that violence against women is a public health problem that needs to be addressed as a socio-political issue and that counselling should be part of the community heath care programme.

A community problem that has differential impacts on women is the issue of Trafficking and Prostitution. Arz has been involved with women in the Baina Beach Red-Light area and they find that the 'phenomenon' of prostitution spares no woman in the community. In the red-light area it affects those in the prostitution trade and also those who are not directly involved. Their case study shows that, intervention and concern can make a difference.

Mariette Correa shows how the proportion of women infected with HIV and AIDS world-wide and also in Goa over the years has been steadily increasing. She says that women in developing countries are much more at risk and explains these vulnerabilities. She concludes with recommendations for action by governments, multilateral agencies and donors etc including the incorporation of gender analysis into HIV/AIDS work at the community level, inter-sectoral collaboration and the integration of rights-based frameworks to address root causes of these vulnerabilities.

One intervention that has been part of the health campaign is sex education. But Sheela Gupte proposes a new approach to combating sexually transmitted diseases, HIV/AIDS and the reduction of teenage abortions. She therefore focuses on adolescent sexuality and is based on her own experiences with this community as a gynaecologist.

Just as prevention is better than cure, detection brings us closer to cure. This is especially true about cervical cancer, which is the second most common form of cancer among women. Eugene D'Silva and Pia Muriel Cardoso propose universal screening for cervical cancer which would identify women at risk for the disease, and enable treatment with pre-cancer cell change thereby reduce the incidence of cervical cancer and mortality from the disease. The cost of such a screening programme is relatively low and therefore an attainable target in Goa.

The right to life is enshrined in the constitution and therefore the provision of health services is a human right of every woman in India. However, this is not an exercised right and Albertina Almeida documents the nature of violations of women's rights to health, in daily experiences in Goa. These violations the author opines are taking place due to the present political economy and highlights the need for a rights approach that will address these concerns.

Just as the provision of health is a right, there are ethical issues involved in the clinical research that is conducted in India by various drug companies who often use women as 'guinea pigs'. Laxmi Murthy argues for monitoring of clinical research by 'independent' bodies, developing effective ways of checking violations of ethical norms and safeguarding the rights, health and well-being of research subjects. She focuses on campaign strategies of the women's health movement both nationally and internationally.

Many argue that issues relating to children cannot be separated from women's issues since in developing countries mothers still bear the major responsibility of child rearing too. Besides, the girl child is the woman of tomorrow. Children's Rights in Goa highlights the vulnerability of the mine workers and focuses on the health of the children whose families are involved in unloading and loading ore and who play an invaluable role in Goa's development. The paper is based on a case study of the children in one mining area in Goa where some children attend the open school run by Children's Rights in Goa.

Fatima da Silva Gracias highlights the vulnerability of the aged and in particular the women in Goa. Her paper is largely based on work that was done the author through the Research Institute for Women on facilities at the homes for the aged in Goa.

Melsa Vas Monteiro provides a deep understanding of the neglected issue of disability and handicap. The list of recommendations for intervention is long which only demonstrates the lacunae that have to be filled.

Bernadette Gomes looks at indigenous health care in Goa which are even now the first remedy sought for minor illnesses. These include 'ganvti vokod' in which women play a lead role which mean providing remedies using plant and animal parts, as also other practices for recovering health like removal of evil eye 'dixtt', driving away evil spirits 'varyachem', trance, penance. It also includes 'Ghorguti vokod' or home remedies. The author talks of the benefits of this system of health care which need to be better documented and researched as it is a dying system of knowledge.

Usha Salelkar shows how the practice of homeopathy which was banned in Goa during the Portuguese rule has proved to serve the health needs of women and children in

Goa by tracing experiences both in government service and private practice, post liberation. This paper is a first hand account of the first Homeopathic Physician to be appointed by the Government of Goa. The paper highlights the merits of homeopathy with a proposal to strengthen homeopathic care in Goa through the government health services to better meet the goals of the Reproductive and Child Health Programme with no big financial cost to the Government of Goa.

## Acknowledgements

I owe my gratitude to all those who made this effort possible and who made working on this exercise enjoyable.

I would like to make a special mention of the Goa State Commission for Women team, particularly Dr. Pramod Salgaonkar, Ex. Chairperson, and Ms. Candida Fernandes, Ex. Member Secretary for their wholehearted support and encouragement and also Ms. Rina Ray, Former Secretary, Women and Child Development and Dr. G.J.S. Abraham, former Dean of Goa Medical College for their involvement with the issue and their suggestions.

# THE CONTRIBUTORS

**Albertina Almeida** is an activist with Bailancho Saad (a Goa-based women's collective) and a practising lawyer.

**Arz** is a Development Organisation, based in the red-light area of Baina Beach, Goa that works to combat trafficking in humans for commercial sexual exploitation.

**Bernadette Gomes** teaches Sociology at the Government College of Arts in Quepem, Goa. Her doctoral work was on indigenous health practices.

**Children's Rights in Goa** is a non-profit organisation that works for children. They have been paticularly active in their campaign against child abuse.

**Eugene D'Silva** [DGO.MD.DNB.MRCOG(London), FRCS(Edin)] is a Consultant Obstetrician and Gynaecologist. He is currently Lecturer with the Department of Obstetrics and Gynaecology, Goa Medical College.

**Fatima da Silva Gracias** teaches History at the Dhempe College of Arts in Goa. Her doctoral work was on the health services in colonial Goa.

**Fiona Dias Saxena** was with the Sangath Society, Goa and is also a professional counsellor.

**Imrana Qadeer** is a Professor and Head of the Centre of Social Medicine and Community Health, Jawaharlal Nehru University, New Delhi. She has also been adviser to the Planning Commission of India.

**Laxmi Murthy** is a journalist and activist with Saheli, Delhi.

**Marcus Hughes** is with the Institute of Psychiatry, Kings College, London, and was on a Wellcome Trust research fellowship at the Sangath Society, Goa.

**Mariette Correa** was the NGO Adviser with the Goa Society for AIDS Control.

**Melsa Vas Monteiro** works for Caritas Goa.

**Nandita de Souza** is a Pediatrician and the Ex-Chairperson of the Sangath Society, Goa.

**Pia Muriel Cardoso** (DGO, MD) is a Senior Resident with the Department of Obstetrics and Gynaecology, Goa Medical College.

**Prabha S. Chandra** is the Additional Professor of Psychiatry, NIMHANS, Bangalore.

**Pradeep Padwal** is the Chief Medical Officer, State Family Welfare Bureau, Directorate of Health Services, Goa.

**Sheela Gupte** is an Obstetrician and Gynaecologist.

**Usha Salelkar** was the Ex. Senior Homeopathic Physician, Directorate of Health Services, Goa and Current Private Homeopathic Practitioner.

**Vikram Patel** is a Senior Lecturer, London School of Hygiene and Tropical Medicine and Chairperson of the Sangath Society, Goa.

# OVERVIEW OF HEALTH POLICY AND PROGRAMME

1

# GENDER AND HEALTH

## Beyond Numbers

*Imrana Qadeer*

'Health' or 'disease', the moment these words are spoken the images of doctors, hospitals laboratories, pathological reports and the causative agents overpower our imagination. That is why I have chosen to address the issue of health from a non-medical perspective of gender. At the very outset therefore, I would like to state that unlike the WHO's definition of health which emphasises the 'state' of well being. I would like to tackle the issue of health as a 'process'. The available quantitative methods however, have limitations in revealing the complex relationships of disease processes. The outcome, the state of well-being, is measured, intervened with and allegedly improved by medical technology. Medical science however, does not fully explain health or disease except in those cases where technology itself is the cause of disease. Such a process has been termed "iatrogenesis" (Illich, 1977). Let me also confess that though I am fully aware of the importance of working towards health, I would, in this paper focus on disease. There is always the danger of succumbing to the biomedical perspective while talking of disease. Yet, I begin with disease for two reasons. Firstly, given the load of morbidity and mortality among women specially the poor women, the struggle for health cannot exclude the challenge of dealing with disease. Secondly, the very construct of 'well being' is a social construct that reflects the social articulation of biological processes—mental, social, and physical. The analysis of the disease process, within a social perspective then, inevitable helps envision well being by exploring social roots of disease as well as the role of technology and desirable changes at both levels.

As we attempt to go beyond numbers, I would like to emphasise that, to do so one needs to look hard at numbers. One needs to understand how statistics acquires new meaning over time by changing definitions, merging categories and generating one kind of data and ignoring the other kind. In the area of women's health such an exercise throws up many interesting insights. However, before we do that, it is important to have our questions and our perspectives clearly worked out. Women's poor health is not only reflected in the gender differentials but also within the differentials across classes and castes. At each level of this socio-economic hierarchy, patriarchy, through inculcating gender inequality around work, sexuality, entitlement, inheritance, access to opportunities and freedom of choice, binds women to roles that are inferior. It tilts the power balance in favour of men.

These unequal relationships between men and women legitimise a range of gender differentials, which vary across caste/class combinations. Gender roles are much more divergent depending upon forms that patriarchy takes and the social process it manifests through. In other words, there is no one articulation of gender and it is not a simple addition to class caste inequalities. For example, issues such as inheritance, entitlements, access to facilities and control over choice may be the key operatives in lower middle and middle classes but their hold lessens among the poor. However, it never vanishes as patriarchal values continue to dominate the mindset irrespective of absence of any significant property that is basic to inheritance and entitlement. For the very rich and educated, though opportunities open up, as do choices, the basic issue of right to property remains.

Other than putting gender in opposition to class and caste, lately the attention has also been shifted from absolute poverty to issues of equity. This is primarily because of the shift in debate from third world problems to the 1st world itself where inequity and not absolute poverty is the major contemporary dilemma. Secondly, the official statistical jugglery has propagated the myth that absolute poverty in India has declined significantly. The reality is that, over the 90s the decline if any has been marginal and serious estimates of poverty vary between 31-34 per cent (Sen, 1999). A big chunk of those lying above the poverty line are only slightly better off as they can barely make ends meet. In other words, almost half the population is extremely vulnerable where women work rigorously to eke out a living.

Poverty also generates extremely unhealthy conditions of environment that are conducive to disease. For example, in rural areas on an average 23.2 per cent population has tap water to drink, *'Pucca'* wells, tube wells and hand pumps provide for 70.8 per cent of the population and 5.4 per cent people depend upon rivers, canals, tanks, ponds and other sources of drinking water. For urban areas these percentages are 73.0, 12.0 and 1.3 per cent. There is no provision for latrines in 84.4 and 23.0 per cent of the rural and urban households respectively. Also, there is total absence of any drainage facility in 62.0 per cent of rural and 20.0 per cent of urban households. This overall picture is problematic enough but, when we see the distribution of these facilities by monthly per capita expenditure (MPCE) groups and social class (SC and ST), the problem compounds itself. When we examine these very services by class and caste, the distribution gets further skewed. For example, among the poorest 20 per cent of the population in rural areas, only 15.4 per cent access tap water. For SC, ST households this proportion is 18 per cent. For the poorest 20 per cent households by MPCE in the urban area, tap water supply is restricted to only per cent as against an average of 73 per cent. Similarly, absence of latrines is reported in 93.4 per cent of the poorest 20 per cent rural and 52.7 per cent urban households. For SC, ST households these respective proportions were 89.0 and 42.0 per cent (See—Tables 1, 2, 3).

These class and caste disadvantages are critical for women's health as women are primarily responsible for

**Table 1:** Per 1000 distribution of households by major source of drinking water

**A:** By MPCE fractile groups

| *State/ UT* | | *Major source of drinking water* | | | | | | | | *Households* | |
|---|---|---|---|---|---|---|---|---|---|---|---|
| | | *Tap* | *Tube well/ hand pump* | *Tan-ker* | *Pucca well* | *Tank/ pond reser-ved for drin-king* | *River/ canal* | *Other* | *Total* | *Estd. (00)* | *Sam-ple* |
| *Fractile group (all-India)* | | | | | | | | | | | |
| 0-10 | R | 154 | 544 | 5 | 233 | 11 | 21 | 30 | 1000 | 100742 | 5668 |
| | U | 586 | 291 | 11 | 92 | 2 | 3 | 14 | 1000 | 33458 | 3830 |
| 10-20 | R | 155 | 539 | 2 | 253 | 10 | 14 | 23 | 1000 | 106261 | 5579 |
| | U | 622 | 267 | 7 | 86 | 2 | 3 | 10 | 1000 | 34671 | 4128 |
| 20-40 | R | 187 | 530 | 2 | 222 | 12 | 16 | 27 | 1000 | 227317 | 12064 |
| | U | 661 | 235 | 10 | 75 | 6 | 2 | 11 | 1000 | 74042 | 8898 |
| 40-60 | R | 233 | 494 | 4 | 211 | 16 | 13 | 25 | 1000 | 243492 | 13056 |
| | U | 737 | 181 | 10 | 56 | 4 | 2 | 8 | 1000 | 83554 | 9575 |
| 60-80 | R | 250 | 475 | 4 | 214 | 16 | 13 | 25 | 1000 | 265505 | 15010 |
| | U | 774 | 163 | 5 | 44 | 3 | 1 | 8 | 1000 | 94549 | 10459 |
| 80-90 | R | 282 | 461 | 4 | 194 | 20 | 11 | 25 | 1000 | 144081 | 8519 |
| | U | 807 | 137 | 6 | 38 | 2 | 1 | 7 | 1000 | 56794 | 6067 |
| 90-100 | R | 311 | 418 | 7 | 218 | 16 | 10 | 20 | 1000 | 175225 | 11388 |
| | U | 845 | 108 | 6 | 29 | 1 | 0 | 9 | 1000 | 67300 | 6701 |

*contd.*

*contd.* ***table 1***

B: By Caste groups

| *State/ UT* | | *Major source of drinking water* | | | | | | | | *Households* | |
|---|---|---|---|---|---|---|---|---|---|---|---|
| | | *Tap* | *Tube well/ hand pump* | *Tanker* | *Pucca well* | *Tank/ pond reserved for drinking* | *River/ canal* | *Other* | *Total* | *Estd. (00)* | *Sample* |
| *Fractile group (all-India)* | | | | | | | | | | | |
| ST | R | 155 | 442 | 4 | 255 | 27 | 47 | 69 | 1000 | 136419 | 12772 |
| | U | 667 | 165 | 10 | 111 | 11 | 5 | 23 | 1000 | 13053 | 3159 |
| SC | R | 209 | 556 | 4 | 190 | 11 | 12 | 15 | 1000 | 290844 | 14311 |
| | U | 658 | 260 | 10 | 50 | 4 | 2 | 16 | 1000 | 64832 | 6634 |
| Other | R | 252 | 475 | 4 | 222 | 14 | 9 | 21 | 1000 | 834713 | 44157 |
| | U | 754 | 172 | 7 | 54 | 3 | 1 | 8 | 1000 | 366366 | 39846 |
| n.r | R | 91 | 469 | – | 172 | 44 | 71 | 1 | 1000 | 647 | 44 |
| | U | 459 | 22 | 14 | 258 | 0 | – | – | 1000 | 116 | 19 |
| All | R | 232 | 490 | 4 | 218 | 15 | 14 | 25 | 1000 | 1262623 | 71284 |
| | U | 737 | 185 | 8 | 55 | 3 | 1 | 9 | 1000 | 444368 | 49658 |
| Estd. 00 no. of households | R | 292780 | 618601 | 5062 | 275198 | 18659 | 173272 | 31698 | 1000 | – | – |
| | U | 327645 | 81995 | 3393 | 24515 | 1403 | 589 | 4060 | 1000 | – | – |
| Sample No. of households | R | 15392 | 31767 | 294 | 15352 | 2235 | 2386 | 3641 | 1000 | – | – |
| | U | 35883 | 8611 | 402 | 3233 | 501 | 149 | 737 | 1000 | – | – |

*Source:* NSS 52nd Round Report no. 445(52/25.0/2), Table A-1, A-2

cleanliness and drinking water supplies for the family. In the process of accomplishing their social roles, they often end up losing their health. The gendered notion of responsibilities and work reflects equally in their contributions through the labour market. Despite their socially productive contributions, they retain a secondary status, both in terms of their participation and wages. This too is reflected in the available statistics.

After the 80s the rise in women's work participation has not been significant. Casualisation has increased with diversification into non-wage activities in labour households with land where self-employment has also risen among women (Kundu, 1999). As a result, earner population ratios in rural

**Table 2:** Per household distribution of households by type of latrine
**A:** By MPCE fractile groups

| *State/ UT* | | *No latrine* | *Type of latrine* | | | | | *Households* | |
|---|---|---|---|---|---|---|---|---|---|
| | | | *Service latrine* | *Septic latrine* | *Flush system* | *Other* | *Total* | *Estd. (00)* | *Sample* |
| *Fractile group (all-India)* | | | | | | | | | |
| 0-10 | R | 944 | 16 | 14 | 2 | 24 | 1000 | 100700 | 5666 |
| | U | 598 | 75 | 203 | 75 | 48 | 1000 | 33456 | 3830 |
| 10-20 | R | 943 | 12 | 8 | 2 | 35 | 1000 | 106309 | 5580 |
| | U | 457 | 87 | 273 | 117 | 66 | 1000 | 34673 | 4128 |
| 20-40 | R | 910 | 19 | 23 | 1 | 47 | 1000 | 227310 | 12065 |
| | U | 360 | 80 | 339 | 161 | 60 | 1000 | 74049 | 8899 |
| 40-60 | R | 876 | 20 | 41 | 4 | 60 | 1000 | 243428 | 13052 |
| | U | 234 | 63 | 418 | 233 | 52 | 1000 | 83542 | 9573 |
| 60-80 | R | 836 | 26 | 64 | 3 | 70 | 1000 | 265572 | 15012 |
| | U | 136 | 45 | 445 | 334 | 40 | 1000 | 94556 | 10461 |
| 80-90 | R | 771 | 34 | 98 | 8 | 89 | 1000 | 143966 | 8520 |
| | U | 88 | 36 | 443 | 405 | 29 | 1000 | 56792 | 6066 |
| 90-100 | R | 669 | 32 | 185 | 24 | 90 | 1000 | 175338 | 11389 |
| | U | 35 | 22 | 341 | 577 | 25 | 1000 | 67300 | 6701 |

*contd.*

*contd.* **table 2**

**B:** By caste groups

| *State/ UT* | | *No latrine* | *Type of latrine* | | | | | *Households* | |
|---|---|---|---|---|---|---|---|---|---|
| | | | *Service latrine* | *Septic latrine* | *Flush system* | *Other* | *Total* | *Estd. (00)* | *Sample* |
| *Fractile group (all-India)* | | | | | | | | | |
| 0-10 | R | 944 | 16 | 14 | 2 | 24 | 1000 | 100700 | 5666 |
| | U | 598 | 75 | 203 | 75 | 48 | 1000 | 33456 | 3830 |
| ST | R | 881 | 25 | 27 | 1 | 66 | 1000 | 136419 | 12772 |
| | U | 427 | 59 | 315 | 135 | 65 | 1000 | 13053 | 3159 |
| SC | R | 909 | 15 | 29 | 3 | 43 | 1000 | 290844 | 14311 |
| | U | 430 | 59 | 262 | 199 | 50 | 1000 | 64832 | 6634 |
| Other | R | 816 | 26 | 82 | 8 | 68 | 1000 | 834713 | 44157 |
| | U | 187 | 54 | 397 | 319 | 43 | 1000 | 366366 | 39846 |
| n.r. | R | 642 | 62 | 48 | – | 96 | 1000 | 647 | 44 |
| | U | 328 | – | 429 | 26 | 6 | 1000 | 116 | 19 |
| all | R | 844 | 23 | 64 | 6 | 62 | 1000 | 1262623 | 71284 |
| | U | 230 | 55 | 375 | 296 | 44 | 1000 | 44368 | 49658 |
| Estd. | R | 1065713 | 29446 | 81029 | 7652 | 78553 | 1000 | – | – |
| (00) no. of house-holds | U | 102184 | 24501 | 166452 | 131336 | 19768 | 1000 | – | – |
| Sample | R | 55025 | 2140 | 3998 | 396 | 9707 | 1000 | – | – |
| No. of house-holds | U | 10674 | 3131 | 18982 | 12959 | 3895 | 1000 | – | – |

*Source:* NSS 52nd Round Report no. 445(52/25.0/2), Table A-4, A-5

labour households show a clear decline. From 41.4 in 1974-75 to 30.3 in 1993-94 among the females as against men, where it has moved from 55.5 to 57.1 over the same period (Papola, 1999). Added to this stagnation is the fact that over the 90s the rise in agricultural wages for women stagnated and those for men actually declined! The non-farm employment also showed similar trends of stagnation in rural areas where women were at a much greater disadvantage due to lower skills, educational qualifications and professional training (Chadha, 1999). They constituted only 15.8 per cent of the total industrial workers in 1996 (Srivastava, 1999).

This failure of the system to adequately absorb the working population evidently impacts women much more. They are not only denied participation but also pushed into the marginalized spaces with poor wages as their men bear the consequences of restricted job opportunities. On the whole, the worker population ratios show 32.8 women per thousand

**Table 3:** Per 1000 distribution of households by type of drainage
**A:** By MPCE fractile groups

| *State/ UT* | | *No drain-age* | *Type of drainage* | | | | | *Households* | |
|---|---|---|---|---|---|---|---|---|---|
| | | | *Open kuccha* | *Open pucca* | *Covered pucca* | *Under ground* | *Total* | *Estd. (00)* | *Sample* |
| *Fractile group (all-India)* | | | | | | | | | |
| 0-10 | R | 693 | 272 | 23 | 6 | 6 | 1000 | 100742 | 5668 |
| | U | 427 | 219 | 260 | 47 | 46 | 1000 | 33458 | 3830 |
| 10-20 | R | 675 | 281 | 31 | 5 | 8 | 1000 | 106261 | 5579 |
| | U | 358 | 205 | 302 | 63 | 73 | 1000 | 34671 | 4128 |
| 20-40 | R | 667 | 273 | 44 | 8 | 8 | 1000 | 227317 | 12064 |
| | U | 285 | 175 | 349 | 106 | 84 | 1000 | 74042 | 8898 |
| 40-60 | R | 637 | 280 | 60 | 13 | 10 | 1000 | 243492 | 13056 |
| | U | 213 | 145 | 392 | 134 | 115 | 1000 | 83554 | 9575 |
| 60-80 | R | 623 | 271 | 81 | 18 | 7 | 1000 | 265505 | 15010 |
| | U | 142 | 101 | 401 | 179 | 177 | 1000 | 94549 | 10459 |
| 80-90 | R | 582 | 276 | 114 | 20 | 7 | 1000 | 144081 | 8519 |
| | U | 113 | 80 | 370 | 204 | 233 | 1000 | 56794 | 6067 |
| 90-100 | R | 543 | 245 | 155 | 37 | 19 | 1000 | 175225 | 11388 |
| | U | 65 | 46 | 272 | 241 | 376 | 1000 | 67300 | 6701 |

*contd.*

*contd.* ***table 3***

**B: By caste groups**

| *State/ UT* | | *No drain-age* | *Type of drainage* | | | | | *Households* | |
|---|---|---|---|---|---|---|---|---|---|
| | | | *Open kuccha* | *Open pucca* | *Covered pucca* | *Under ground* | *Total* | *Estd. (00)* | *Sample* |
| *Fractile group (all-India)* | | | | | | | | | |
| ST | R | 784 | 187 | 26 | 1 | 1 | 1000 | 136419 | 12772 |
| | U | 377 | 145 | 306 | 76 | 96 | 1000 | 13053 | 3159 |
| SC | R | 644 | 288 | 51 | 7 | 10 | 1000 | 290844 | 14311 |
| | U | 314 | 172 | 317 | 77 | 121 | 1000 | 64832 | 6634 |
| Other | R | 597 | 279 | 92 | 22 | 11 | 1000 | 834713 | 44157 |
| | U | 176 | 119 | 356 | 168 | 180 | 1000 | 366366 | 39846 |
| n.r. | R | 279 | 526 | 32 | 11 | - | 1000 | 647 | 44 |
| | U | 362 | 128 | 206 | 93 | - | 1000 | 116 | 19 |
| all | R | 628 | 271 | 75 | 16 | 9169 | 1000 | 1262623 | 71284 |
| | U | 202 | 128 | 349 | 152 | 169 | 1000 | 444368 | 49658 |
| Estd. (00) | R | 792634 | 342350 | 95251 | 20276 | 11878 | 1000 | – | – |
| No. of house-holds | U | 89837 | 56674 | 155011 | 67557 | 75142 | 1000 | – | – |
| Sample | R | 47430 | 18023 | 4529 | 767 | 506 | 1000 | – | – |
| No. of house-holds | U | 11220 | 6979 | 17755 | 6485 | 7199 | 1000 | – | – |

*Source:* NSS 52nd Round Report No. 445(52/25.0/2), Tables A-7, A-8.

population as against 553 men per thousand population in rural areas for the year 1993-94. For urban areas these ratios are 155 and 521 respectively for the same year (Sundaram, 2001). For 2001, these values for women have come down to 30. This economic "incapability" and the lack of skill are again a function of women's prescribed social role. The differentials in the patterns of displacement, be it casualisation or shift out from wage earning jobs, are not uniform in different classes but gender specific. These reflect the underlying dynamics of gender in determining work and wage differentials in labouring populations. Despite all these evidences of the interdependence of class, caste and gender, the present tendency in health research is to focus on gender alone and explain away differences in health of men and women as out come of this social construct alone. This paper emphasises the role of the inter linkages.

To explore the relevance of this triad (caste, per cent class and gender), we propose to first look at the available data on mortality and morbidity and women's access to services to explore the dynamic of health and disease. Then we examine the limits of simplified gender analysis for health issues and its implications for policy and programmes.

## Class, Caste, Gender and Patterns of Mortality, Morbidity and Service Utilisation

The existing divide between the rich and poor that gets lost in national averages has been captured by through poor—rich mortality ratios in developing countries (Gwatkin, 2001). He uses mortality in the poorest 10 to 20 per cent of population as a multiple of the mortality in the richest 10 to 20 per cent population. These ratios are highest in the higher income developing countries (fifteen times higher in 1-4 year age group and 6 times till 29 year of age). Among the lower income countries these ratios are not as high though they are above one. Similarly, these ratios are highest for pregnancy complications, infectious diseases and perinatal conditions. Countries studies were sub-Sahara Asian and Latin American.

It needs to be stated straight away that the available data on these relationships is far from satisfactory. Most national sources of statistics neglect the issue of stratification and despite records keep silent on class-wise analysis of data. A 1989 publication of the government's Vital Statistics Division, happened to provide some key tables that are reproduced here (See—Tables 4, 5, 6, 7). Though the vital statistics department has not repeated this exercise since then, it can be assumed that the caste, class differentials continue to be a part of the present mortality scenario, as the income differentials have only increased over the 90s and absolute poverty has declined only marginally. Added to this differential is the fact of a declining sex ratio in the age group 0-6 years, in 577 districts, despite a slightly improved overall sex ratio (from 927 in 1991to 933 in 2001). The number of districts with normal sex ratio (1000-1049), are only 8 covering 0.38 per cent of the total population. In 239 districts, sex ratio ranges from 950-999 and the districts have 39 per cent of the total population. The remaining 330 districts have ratios under 950 and 16 of them have a ratio of less than 800 (GoI, 2001). These gender differentials continue to prevail for women in reproductive age group. The respite is visible only in the older age group and in those between 6 to 12 years of age.

**Table 4:** IMR by level of income

| *Annual Households Income* | *Rural* | *Urban* | *Comb.* |
|---|---|---|---|
| 5000 and below | 128.6 | 85.4 | 124.2 |
| 5001 - 10,000 | 108.1 | 71.5 | 100.7 |
| 10,001 and above | 91.8 | 51.5 | 79.7 |

*Source:* Govt. of India, Vital Statistics Dept. 1985.

**Table 5:** MR by SC/ Tribe Status of women

| *Caste* | *Rural* | *Urban* | *Comb.* |
|---|---|---|---|
| Scheduled Caste | 131.7 | 92.9 | 126.5 |
| Scheduled Tribe | 103.2 | 67.7 | 101.1 |
| Non-scheduled Caste/Tribe | 110.0 | 62.5 | 91.2 |

*Source:* Govt. of India, Vital Statistics Dept. 1985

**Table 6:** Estimated death rates for broad age groups by total annual income of the household - India, 1984.

| *Broad age group* | *Annual Income (Rs. )* | | |
|---|---|---|---|
| | *Rs. 5,000 and below* | *5,001 - 10,000* | *10,000 and above* |
| | | RURAL | |
| 0-4 | 52.4 | 4.8 | 34.0 |
| 5-14 | 5.1 | 3.8 | 2.9 |
| 15-34 | 4.4 | 2.8 | 2.3 |
| 35-49 | 8.0 | 4.9 | 3.8 |
| 50- | 46.4 | 37.7 | 33.1 |
| All ages | 16.9 | 12.6 | 10.7 |
| | | URBAN | |
| 0-4 | 33.2 | 24.4 | 16.6 |
| 5-14 | 3.9 | 2.4 | 1.4 |
| 15-34 | 3.8 | 2.3 | 1.4 |
| 35-49 | 10.1 | 5.1 | 3.0 |
| 50- | 45.9 | 36.0 | 29.0 |
| All ages | 14.0 | 9.0 | 6.5 |
| | | COMBINED | |
| 0-4 | 50.3 | 37.9 | 28.3 |
| 5-14 | 5.0 | 3.5 | 2.4 |
| 15-34 | 4.3 | 2.7 | 2.0 |
| 35-49 | 8.2 | 4.9 | 3.5 |
| 50- | 46.4 | 37.4 | 31.7 |
| All ages | 16.6 | 11.8 | 9.1 |

*Source:* Govt. of India, Office of the Register General (1984).

**Table 7:** Death Rates Age groups by Total annual Income Estimated death rates for age groups by Scheduled Caste/ Tribes status—India, 1984

| *Broad age group* | *Scheduled Caste (SC)* | *Scheduled Tribe (ST)* | *Non-SC/ ST* |
|---|---|---|---|
| | | RURAL | |
| 0-4 | 54.9 | 46.5 | 40.9 |
| 5-14 | 5.7 | 5.0 | 3.6 |
| 15-34 | 4.0 | 4.1 | 3.0 |
| 35-49 | 6.8 | 8.3 | 5.4 |
| 50- | 45.9 | 41.7 | 38.7 |
| All ages | 17.0 | 15.0 | 12.9 |
| | | URBAN | |
| 0-4 | 33.0 | 25.6 | 21.0 |
| 5-14 | 3.3 | 3.1 | 2.0 |
| 15-34 | 2.8 | 3.1 | 2.0 |
| 35-49 | 7.0 | 6.6 | 4.6 |
| 50- | 42.5 | 44.6 | 33.5 |
| All ages | 11.6 | 10.7 | 8.2 |
| | | COMBINED | |
| 0-4 | 51.6 | 45.0 | 36.0 |
| 5-14 | 5.3 | 4.9 | 3.3 |
| 15-34 | 3.8 | 4.0 | 2.7 |
| 35-49 | 6.8 | 8.2 | 5.2 |
| 50- | 45.5 | 41.9 | 37.5 |
| All ages | 16.2 | 14.7 | 11.7 |

*Source:* Govt. of India Office of the Register General (1984)

When we look at the causes of these deaths, those due to pregnancy related problems and diseases of blood and blood forming organs are higher in women and the diseases of circulatory system are higher in men. Percentages of deaths due to various other causes are almost similar (See—Table 8).

**Table 8:** Survey of Causes of Death (Rural) Percentage Distribution of Deaths as per International Classification of Diseases—10th Revision All India (Rural )—1995.

*(in percentage)*

| *Code No.* | *Probable Cause of Death* | *M* | *F* | *P* |
|---|---|---|---|---|
| A | Infection and Parasitic Diseases | 12.7 | 11.0 | 11.9 |
| B | Viral Infection | 4.5 | 5.0 | 4.7 |
| C | Neoplasm | 3.8 | 4.6 | 4.2 |
| D | Diseases of the Blood and Blood Forming Organs | 2.5 | 3.6 | 3.0 |
| E | Metabolic Diseases | 1.0 | 0.8 | 0.9 |
| F | Mental and Behavioural Disorders | 0.4 | 0.5 | 0.5 |
| G | Inflammatory Diseases of Central Nervous System | 4.9 | 4.5 | 4.8 |
| I | Diseases of Circulatory System | 10.8 | 7.9 | 9.5 |
| J | Diseases of the Respiratory System | 16.7 | 16.5 | 16.6 |
| K | Diseases of the Digestive System | 2.0 | 1.1 | 1.6 |
| N | Diseases of the Genitourinary System | 0.9 | 0.5 | 0.7 |
| O | Pregnancy of Childbirth and Puerperium | 0.0 | 1.9 | 0.8 |
| P | Conditions of Originating in the Perinatal Period | 8.7 | 9.7 | 9.2 |
| Q | Congenital Malformations Deformations and Abnormalities | 0.3 | 0.3 | 0.3 |
| R | Symptoms Signs and Abnormal Clinical Finding not elsewhere mention | 17.2 | 20.3 | 18.6 |
| T | Injuries Poisoning and other Consequences of External Causes | 0.8 | 2.2 | 1.4 |
| V | External Causes of Mortality | 3.3 | 1.3 | 2.4 |
| W | Other External Causes of Accidental Injuries | 0.6 | 0.4 | 0.5 |
| X | With Venomous Animal Contact other Medically | 6.5 | 5.4 | 6.0 |
|  | Certified Deaths | 2.3 | 2.5 | 2.4 |
|  | Grand Total | 100.00 | 100.00 | 100.00 |

*Source:* Survey of Causes of Death (Rural), Govt. of India, Survey of causes of Death 1996.

When we review the prevailing patterns of nutritional status, we find that there are distinct differences between different occupational classes. The agricultural labour households and marginal farmers have the highest levels of protein calorie deficiencies (See—Table 9). The National Nutrition Monitoring Bureau data thus provides evidence of relatively poorer nutritional status as we go down the occupational class hierarchy.

**Table 9:** Estimates of Percentage distribution of household by Protein, Calorie Adequacy Status by Occupation

| *Occupation* | *P C* | *P C* | *P C* | *P C* | *Estimates* | |
|---|---|---|---|---|---|---|
| *Marginal* | - - | - + | + + | + - | *Prot. Inadequacy* | *Calorie Inadequacy* |
| Farmers | 17.1 | 0.9 | 48.6 | 33.4 | 18.0 | 50.5 |
| Small Farmers | 9.9 | - | 65.0 | 25.1 | 9.9 | 35.0 |
| Large Farmers | 14.0 | - | 60.7 | 25.3 | 1.0 | 39.3 |
| Agr. Labour | 20.0 | 0.3 | 46.9 | 32.8 | 20.0 | 52.8 |
| Others | 15.7 | - | 55.9 | 28.4 | 15.7 | 44.1 |

*Source:* NNMB, Report 1996.

The available national data thus reveals caste and class differentials as well as gender differentials in mortality that reflects a bias against women through increasing numbers of missing girls. What it does not reveal however is the gender differentials within classes or the distribution of classes within varying ranges of sex ratios. Going by the sex ratio differentials, it can be said without hesitation that there is no linear relationship between class and gender differentials in mortality. This is indicated by the fact that the ten districts with the lowest sex ratios are located in the economically advanced States of Punjab and Haryana (GoI, 2001). Given the limited scope of analysis of the national data by the vital statistics and sample Registration Schemes, we also examined the morbidity statistics provided by the National Sample Survey. Here too we faced problems though of a very different nature.

Other than total morbidity in MPCE groups, NSS also provides data on caste related morbidity. Compared to the average reported morbidity, the SC, ST groups have very high reported morbidity. The average reported morbidity among women is higher both in rural and urban areas. This gender differential is higher for acute diseases as compared to the chronic diseases (See Table 10A, 10B). When this differential for acute and chronic diseases is examined across MPCE groups, the pattern that emerges is interesting. The reported acute and chronic morbidity increases in both sexes with rise in expenditure across rural and urban areas. The increase however is more among women. For the poorest

**Table 10A:** Number of Persons Reporting Ailments: During the last 15 days per 1000 persons by MPCE groups

| | Acute | | | | | | | | | |
|---|---|---|---|---|---|---|---|---|---|---|
| Rural | 1 | 2 | 3 | 4 | 5 | 6 | 7 | All | ST | SC |
| Male | 34 | 32 | 36 | 41 | 43 | 49 | 55 | 41 | 37 | 41 |
| Female | 33 | 33 | 40 | 45 | 47 | 53 | 57 | 44 | 38 | 43 |
| Difference | -1 | +1 | +4 | +4 | +4 | +4 | +2 | +3 | +1 | +2 |
| Person | 34 | 32 | 38 | 43 | 45 | 51 | 56 | 42 | 38 | 42 |
| Urban | | | | | | | | | | |
| Male | 34 | 34 | 37 | 39 | 38 | 40 | 48 | 39 | 35 | 39 |
| Female | 33 | 39 | 42 | 42 | 46 | 54 | 45 | 43 | 37 | 45 |
| Difference | -1 | +5 | +5 | +3 | +8 | +11 | -3 | +4 | +2 | +6 |
| Person | 34 | 37 | 30 | 40 | 42 | 45 | 47 | 41 | 36 | 42 |

*Source:* Govt. of India, NSS 52nd Round, 1995-96

**Table 10B:** Number of Persons Reporting Ailments: During the last 15 days per 1000 persons by MPCE groups.

| | **Chronic** | | | | | | | | | |
|---|---|---|---|---|---|---|---|---|---|---|
| *Rural* | 1 | 2 | 3 | 4 | 5 | 6 | 7 | All | ST | SC |
| Male | 9 | 8 | 9 | 9 | 14 | 17 | 29 | 13 | 5 | 12 |
| Female | 8 | 7 | 9 | 11 | 15 | 20 | 34 | 14 | 5 | 12 |
| Difference | –1 | +1 | 0 | +2 | +1 | +3 | +5 | +1 | 0 | 0 |
| Person | 9 | 7 | 9 | 10 | 14 | 18 | 31 | 13 | 5 | 12 |
| *Urban* | | | | | | | | | | |
| Male | 8 | 8 | 9 | 11 | 13 | 18 | 23 | 13 | 7 | 10 |
| Female | 7 | 9 | 12 | 13 | 18 | 25 | 26 | 15 | 10 | 12 |
| Difference | –1 | +1 | +3 | +2 | +5 | +7 | +3 | +2 | +3 | +2 |
| Person | 8 | 8 | 11 | 12 | 15 | 21 | 24 | 14 | 8 | 11 |

*Source:* Govt. of India, NSS 52nd Round, 1995-96

expenditure groups, in fact the reported morbidity from women is lower than men across rural and urban areas. As we move up towards higher expenditure groups, the reported morbidity in women increases though the increase is much less for chronic diseases. Also, going by the reported illnesses, the women in urban areas seem to be much worse off in better expenditure groups.

This direct relationship between class and illness reporting no doubt reflects a social bias in the process of reporting itself. Reporting is a function of people's perception of the nature of illness. Many not so minor illnesses are considered normal by the poor and not reported. The relative importance of illness and other stresses of survival and access to services and its experience also influence reporting. In contrast however, the higher mortality rates in low-income groups are indicative of higher load of morbidity. Tables 6, 7 strengthen the probability of reporting bias in lower MPCE groups and a likely concentration of illness among the poor. It is for this reason that simply showing a negative class gradient or gender bias against women does not help grasp the nature of the problem. The real issue is to look at disease in relation to the load of poverty and its dynamics. The fact that because the class and gender inequalities are not congruent in terms of how they work (Sen *et al.*, 2002), also does not justify their separate analysis.

Looking at the gender differentials for specific diseases, the NSS presents a clear bias against women for acute diseases like tetanus, fevers, diseases of the eyes, bronchitis and mouth, teeth and gum diseases (See—Table 11). Similarly, the key chronic illnesses more prevalent among women are anemia, sexually transmitted diseases, joint pains, chronic gastric problems and the diseases of the eyes and ears (NSS, 1998). As seen earlier, the over all burden of diseases is heavier for women (See—Table 10). NSS does not provide an MPCE group based analysis for specific diseases though, as we have presented earlier, they do indicate a relatively higher over all reported morbidity for SC's and ST's.

**Table 11:** Incidence of acute ailments per 100,000 person by Age

| S.No. | *Ailments* | | *0-14* | *15-39* | *40-59* | *60 and Above* |
|---|---|---|---|---|---|---|
| 1 | Diarrhoea and Gastroenteritis | M | 361 | 121 | 285 | 664 |
| | | F | 353 | 196 | 209 | 339 |
| 2 | Tetanus | M | 0 | 1 | 3 | - |
| | | F | 10 | 0 | 1 | 4 |
| 3 | Diptheria | M | 9 | 4 | 4 | 0 |
| | | F | 1 | 6 | - | 3 |
| 4 | Whooping Cough | M | 51 | 57 | 57 | 289 |
| | | F | 41 | 37 | 47 | 166 |
| 5 | Meningitic Encephalitis | M | 5 | 1 | 2 | 14 |
| | | F | 2 | 9 | 1 | 0 |
| 6 | Fevers (Short) | M | 2187 | 1153 | 1466 | 2104 |
| | | F | 1955 | 1374 | 1644 | 2555 |
| 7 | Chickenpox | M | 84 | 7 | 1 | 6 |
| | | F | 52 | 13 | 9 | 13 |
| 8 | Measles | M | 28 | 11 | 0 | 11 |
| | | F | 17 | 1 | 2 | 0 |
| 9 | Mumps | M | 5 | 6 | 0 | 0 |
| | | F | 8 | 6 | 0 | 0 |
| 10 | Diseases of the eye | M | 36 | 40 | 34 | 74 |
| | | F | 61 | 29 | 19 | 155 |
| 11 | Acute ear | M | 31 | 10 | 6 | 20 |
| | | F | 21 | 23 | 4 | 0 |
| 12 | Heart failure | M | 2 | 1 | 8 | 39 |
| | | F | 0 | 5 | 2 | 0 |
| 13 | Cerebral Stroke | M | 0 | 3 | 0 | 1 |
| | | F | 0 | 2 | 1 | 2 |
| 14 | Cough/ Bronchitis | M | 191 | 103 | 235 | 595 |
| | | F | 195 | 155 | 224 | 779 |
| 15 | Acute Resp. Inf. + Pneumonia | M | 60 | 11 | 46 | 58 |
| | | F | 51 | 13 | 20 | 85 |
| 16 | Mouth, Teeth and Gum diseases | M | 24 | 18 | 14 | 61 |
| | | F | 35 | 40 | 88 | 37 |
| 17 | Injuries and accidents | M | 77 | 64 | 113 | 102 |
| | | F | 0 | 54 | 9 | 0 |
| 18 | Others up to 30 days | M | 399 | 277 | 426 | 743 |
| | | F | 27 | 30 | 58 | 217 |
| 19 | Undiagnosed | M | 611 | 39 | 61 | 146 |
| | | F | 67 | 60 | 142 | 78 |
| 20 | Short diarrhoea Total | M | 3611 | 1925 | 2760 | 4927 |
| | | F | 3223 | 2474 | 3204 | 5291 |

*Source:* NSS 52nd Round, Report No. 445, 1995-96.

The data on untreated morbidity in contrast to average morbidity shows a negative relationship between morbidity prevalence and increasing MPCE. This is indicative of poor access to services for the most disadvantaged and their inability to avail of it. The decline in untreated morbidity with rising expenditure in families is not only directly linked to economic status but is also gender related. As in reported morbidity, gender differences sharpen with rise in monthly per capita expenditure. This trend perhaps reveals the dialectical relationship between class and gender. While incomes bring relief, it is distributed unequally between sexes and only in the highest expenditure groups there may be some relief for women (See—Table 12).

This somewhat incomplete macro level evidence of links between key social processes and disease, calls for a more rigorous analysis. Instead of searching for the missing evidence or generating it, two kinds of short cuts are used. Either the two sets of influences are examined separately, or, due to paucity of evidence, class and caste differentials are ignored and only gender differentials highlighted. In doing so, we miss on understanding the very processes that determine disease occurrence and women's access to medical care. Invariably, the discussion becomes focused on reproductive health. This is a tactical diversion as it suits the current shifts in policy.

There are very few micro studies that actually try to link class and gender effectively. Where they do so, reported morbidity acquires a very different profile. This is so because extracting information on diseases from women requires time, rapport, patience and an understanding of their hesitations and language. These methodological sophistications cannot be a part of large-scale surveys such as the NSS. Two such studies from Birbhum district of West Bengal and Allahabad district of Uttar Pradesh provide sufficient evidence of links between disease loads and poverty and the gender biases that favour men in each class (Soman, 1992; Malobika, 1993). These studies are indicative of the need for appropriate morbidity studies to correct the impressions created by the macro level data.

**Table 12:** Rates of Untreated Ailments*: All India Trends number untreated per 1000 ailing

| | *Rural* | | | *Urban* | | | *Rural : Urban Ratio* | |
|---|---|---|---|---|---|---|---|---|
| **Gender** | | | | | | | | |
| Male | 172.4 | 162 | -6% | 98.1 | 90 | -8% | 1.76 | 1.80 |
| Female | 198.0 | 184 | -7% | 118.9 | 97 | -18% | 1.67 | 1.90 |
| Both | 184.8 | 173 | -6% | 108.6 | 93 | -14% | 1.70 | 1.86 |
| Female/ Male | 1.15 | 1.14 | -1% | 1.21 | 1.08 | -11% | | |
| Ratio | | | | | | | | |
| MPCE Fractiles* | | | | | | | | |
| **Males** | | | | | | | | |
| 0 to 10 | 198.2 | 276 | 39% | [illegible]11.8 | 180 | 61% | 1.77 | 1.53 |
| 10 to 20 | 175.6 | 210 | 20% | 103.6 | 122 | 18% | 1.70 | 1.72 |
| 20 to 40 | 192.5 | 175 | -9% | 103.1 | 91 | -12% | 1.87 | 1.92 |
| 40 to 60 | 172.8 | 170 | -2% | 88.6 | 80 | -10% | 1.95 | 2.13 |
| 60 to 80 | 167.9 | 162 | -4% | 91.8 | 72 | -22% | 1.83 | 2.25 |
| 80 to 90 | 141.7 | 132 | -7% | 92.5 | 38 | -59% | 1.53 | 3.47 |
| 90 to 100 | 103.6 | 85 | -18% | 122.6 | 102 | -17% | 0.85 | 0.83 |
| Range | 94.6 | 191.0 | | -10.8 | 78.0 | | | |
| **Females** | | | | | | | | |
| 0 to 10 | 233.9 | 241 | 3% | 190.5 | 193 | 1% | 1.23 | 1.25 |
| 10 to 20 | 267.7 | 245 | -8% | 137.0 | 137 | 0% | 1.95 | 1.79 |
| 20 to 40 | 198.1 | 217 | 10% | 128.7 | 105 | -18% | 1.54 | 2.07 |
| 40 to 60 | 207.0 | 206 | 0% | 126.4 | 95 | -25% | 1.64 | 2.17 |
| 60 to 80 | 194.7 | 177 | -9% | 71.4 | 82 | 15% | 2.73 | 2.16 |
| 80 to 90 | 138.6 | 148 | 7% | 90.0 | 54 | -40% | 1.54 | 2.74 |
| 90 to 100 | 92.8 | 106 | 14% | 93.6 | 67 | -28% | 0.99 | 1.58 |
| Range | 141.2 | 135.0 | | 96.9 | 126.0 | | | |

*Source:* Rates of Untreated Ailments* : All India Trends.
1986-87 (NSSO 1992, Statement 11, p. 66) 1995-96 (NSSO 1998, Table 8.2, A-46, A-151).

**Reproductive Health**

In 1994 the UN Conference on Population and Development picked up the notion of reproductive rights and health from the women's movement and located it strictly within the boundaries of Structural Adjustment Policies (SAP). The concept of gender was liberally flouted as it helped highlight reproductive health of women (ICPD, 1994). Issues of class (or caste), political economy and specificity of the Third World nations were kept out of the debate. In absence of any alternative social and economic strategies, reproductive rights and empowerment of women became the central objective, irrespective of structural constraints. Fertility control and women's right over it were pushed to the fore without linking them with her right to dignity, work, education, health and freedom. At the same time focus on male sterilizations declined and HIV, AIDS, STD and RTI acquired the place of priority in morbidity management.

Reproductive health that focused on women's control over their bodies, was seen in the women's movement as a part of the broader agenda of empowerment of all women. Under the presently prevailing circumstances it became an instrument of shifting focus of fertility control from men to women. At the policy level, from safe motherhood reproductive health shifted attention to contraception, RTI, STD and AIDS and remained confined to the reproductive age group (GoI, 1992). It neither linked reproductive health to general health issues, nor highlighted class, caste differentials and the importance of livelihood and survival issues in a milieu where casualisation, decline in work opportunities and dwindling real wages were threatening the working classes.

The funding agencies used gender concerns to promote fertility control through strategic focus on women. It is not surprising then that, reproductive health strategy became the main plank of India's Family Welfare Programme and organisations such as the World Bank, Ford Foundation, USAID, UNFPA, WHO, ODA etc., fully supported it. Even the National Population Policy of 2000, that linked population control strategies to social and economic development and well-being in principle (it saw improved nutrition and control of communicable diseases as key components of its strategy), failed to provide adequate guidelines for action. The result was that States used its loopholes and in the name of a gender sensitive approach, made women their targets (Rao, 2002). Uttar Pradesh for example, despite evidence of harmful effects of hormonal contraceptives (Richter, 1993; Sathyamala, 2000), proposes to include these contraceptives that were earlier rejected by the National Family Planning Programme itself! Women's groups have been protesting against unethical contraceptive research practices for long (Gupta, 2000) but to no avail.

It is worthwhile remembering that pregnancy related mortality today is only 1.9 per cent of total mortality among women. The pattern of illness among pregnant women is the same as that of the young and the unmarried. Pregnancy only enhances pre-existing problems (Sagar, 2001). Thirdly, pregnancy and related factors contribute 15 per cent and communicable diseases and anaemia 35 per cent of the deaths among women of reproductive age group. The latter two constitute 45 per cent of the deaths in the age group 0-14 years (Qadeer, 1998). These trends, when seen in the light of mortality distribution over classes, indicate that for reproductive illness too, the women of the poor and the socially deprived groups would be the main sufferers. The maternal mortality estimates today continue to be as high as 540. The latest NFHS Survey puts the range to 428 to 653 per 100,000 live-births (IIPS, 1999). This survey has attempted to develop a standard of living index (SLI) based on assets. According to this classification, reproductive morbidity such as vaginal discharge with itching and irritation, bad odour, severe lower abdomen pain, fever and other symptoms is definitely higher in the low (SLI) group and low in those with high SLI (See Table 13). A similar higher load is seen among schedule castes and tribes compared to backward classes (IIPS, 1999). In other words this data again emphasises the importance of social and economic linkages of gender deprivation.

**Table 13 :** Currently married women reporting painful intercourse or bleeding alter course by selected background characteristics, India, 1998-99

| *Background characteristic* | *Any abnormal vaginal discharge* | *Itching or irritation* | *Bad odour* | *Severe lower abdominal pain* | *Fever* | *Other problem* | *Sympt toms of urinary tract infection* | *Any abnormal vaginal discharge or symptoms of urinary tract infection* | *Number of every married women* | *Painful inter course (often)* | *Bleeding after inter course (ever)* | *Any reproductive health problem* | *Number of currently married women* |
|---|---|---|---|---|---|---|---|---|---|---|---|---|---|
| | | | | | | *Standard living index* | | | | | | | |
| Low | 31.3 | 17.3 | 12.8 | 20.7 | 9.6 | 8.1 | 19.5 | 37.4 | 29.033 | 13.5 | 2.5 | 41.3 | 26.505 |
| Medium | 30.5 | 17.7 | 11.5 | 18.9 | 8.4 | 8.3 | 18.0 | 36.3 | 41.289 | 13.0 | 2.3 | 40.1 | 38.999 |
| High | 25.6 | 15.3 | 8.7 | 14.5 | 5.0 | 7.0 | 13.7 | 30.6 | 17.845 | 10.1 | 1.7 | 34.0 | 17.173 |

*Source:* NFHS, 1997-98.

Our analysis till now shows that while the class/caste inequalities in health are accepted, its links with reproductive health and the social basis of reproductive health itself has been ignored. While at the policy level a gendered approach has been used to bring women center-stage for the purpose of fertility control, within the academia, a gendered vision of health has meant either highlighting exclusive problems of women arising out of their bondage to patriarchal families (such as violence, mental illnesses or reproductive illnesses), or, focusing on empowering strategies where-in, the rights approach is used to mobilize women to break their intra familial bondage. Both these approaches ignore the vast quantity of diseases of women caused by poverty and deprivation as well as the importance of social institutions and extra familial support structures necessary for empowerment. We are not arguing that violence, mental illness and reproductive problems are less important. We are only pointing out that these problems—like general illnesses—are rooted in the social process. They cannot be dealt with purely technologically as they are a part of the total public health problem and need systemic handling through social policies. Policies that help medical care services contribute to problem management rather than take over the task of prevention. It is wrong to add to the health system's task challenges that are essentially social in nature. Instead of clearly articulating the role that health professionals and heath systems should play in the case of these illnesses (such as diagnosis, supportive role and therapeutic inputs), identifying them purely as health problems contributes to their medicalisation and not necessarily better management.

In fact, those who were earlier pushing reproductive health approach have now shifted to the new domain of addressing inequalities. The approach remains technological, rationalising privatisation of services as well as the retreat of the state and propagating the agenda of self-help. For example, within the framework of SAP, many have accepted the inevitability of a public private mix in services and are busy rationalising it by suggesting controls over the private sectors. They fail to address the basic contradictions between public health and private sector interests. Hence, they have no solutions for the emerging irrational trends in medical practice such as the rising trend of Caesarian sections. Nor do they address the problem of preventing communicable diseases, the neglect of anaemia and under-nutrition that enhance the problem of reproductive health and its complications (Qadeer, 2001). Even the glaring inequalities of access to much proclaimed RCH services (as reflected in differential registration and antenatal care and place of child birth) and professional help (as reflected by type of medical attention), are side lined in planning when the data is provided by the government's own sources (See—Tables 14, 15, 16). Those pushing for the social capital approach over-look the simple fact that for poor people to support each other, a minimum subsistence is required and the very notion of social capital assumes that this minimum exists.

These approaches therefore leave the basic question unanswered. Can structural constraints within third world remain unchallenged before women are empowered or equity in health achieved? The quiet shift from the radical concept of equality of opportunity to equity (fair distribution of basic minimum requirements) within the prevailing system—so that *status quo* is maintained—is too obvious to go unnoticed. It is this need to address the politics and social dynamics of health that a gendered approach should emphasise. Gender obviously is a basic unity of politics itself.

**Policy Implications**

Our analysis primarily points out that to go beyond numbers and statistics we have to first critique our conceptual framework with which we are approaching the available statistics. Only then can we assess the limits of data and define our own directions to move forward. To understand women's health in its totality, the importance of socio-economic and gender inequalities cannot be understated. Most important is the

**Table 14 :** Number of pregnant women registered for pre-natal care per 1000 women (aged 15-49 years), average number of times attended and their per 1000 distribution by reason for seeking pre-natal care.

| State/UT | | No registered per 1000 pregnant women | Ave. No. of times attended | Reason for seeking pre-natal care | | | | | Pregnant women | | | |
|---|---|---|---|---|---|---|---|---|---|---|---|---|
| | | | | Routine pre-natal care | Felt ill | ANW/ LHV advised | Other | Total | Regd. | All | Regd. | All |
| *Fractile group (All-India)* | | | | | | | | | | | | |
| 0-10 | R | 313 | 3.8 | 478 | 71 | 403 | 27 | 1000 | 9687 | 30916 | 863 | 2585 |
| | U | 429 | 4.2 | 757 | 65 | 107 | 45 | 1000 | 2962 | 6909 | 709 | 1472 |
| 10-20 | R | 351 | 4 | 510 | 78 | 344 | 62 | 1000 | 9300 | 26480 | 854 | 2200 |
| | U | 537 | 4.1 | 793 | 57 | 94 | 41 | 1000 | 3486 | 6495 | 838 | 1435 |
| 20-40 | R | 387 | 3.6 | 563 | 55 | 331 | 36 | 1000 | 19479 | 50291 | 1776 | 4256 |
| | U | 636 | 4.4 | 807 | 49 | 70 | 55 | 1000 | 7650 | 12021 | 1810 | 2733 |
| 40-60 | R | 389 | 4.2 | 625 | 68 | 246 | 39 | 1000 | 18446 | 47389 | 1745 | 4021 |
| | U | 714 | 5 | 809 | 54 | 68 | 48 | 1000 | 7525 | 10546 | 1831 | 2443 |
| 60-80 | R | 446 | 4.5 | 678 | 84 | 183 | 41 | 1000 | 19750 | 44237 | 1881 | 3888 |
| | U | 746 | 5.3 | 823 | 59 | 54 | 52 | 1000 | 6696 | 8982 | 1739 | 2169 |
| 80-90 | R | 514 | 4.6 | 686 | 92 | 186 | 24 | 1000 | 10485 | 20401 | 997 | 1853 |
| | U | 762 | 6.2 | 841 | 49 | 75 | 27 | 1000 | 3189 | 4185 | 869 | 1040 |
| 90-100 | R | 605 | 4.7 | 723 | 70 | 145 | 42 | 1000 | 9519 | 15728 | 1059 | 1746 |
| | U | 841 | 6.5 | 842 | 38 | 33 | 70 | 1000 | 3110 | 3696 | 748 | 850 |
| All | R | 411 | 4.2 | 613 | 73 | 259 | 38 | 1000 | 96667 | 235442 | 9175 | 20549 |
| | U | 655 | 5 | 811 | 53 | 69 | 49 | 1000 | 34619 | 52834 | 8544 | 12142 |

*Source:* NSS 52nd Round, Report No. 445, 1995-96, Tables A-89, A-90.

realisation that these social processes cannot be separated and must be dealt with as an entity. Once this is accepted the problems of the present policies for women's health become evident.

Oriented primarily to control population, these policies reflect a unique construction of women. They are either seen as mothers and caretakers or as instruments of fertility control. In the name of empowerment, equity and gender sensitivity, their specific needs are highlighted and the right to reproductive health becomes central. Right to over all good health, education,

**Table 15 :** Per 1000 distribution of mothers by place of childbirth.

| *Fractile group (All-India)* | | *Place of childbirth* | | | | *Number of mothers* | |
|---|---|---|---|---|---|---|---|
| | | *Home* | *Hospital* | *Other* | *Total** | *Estd. (00)* | *Sample* |
| 0-10 | R | 903 | 60 | 8 | 1000 | 25478 | 2358 |
| | U | 615 | 354 | 7 | 1000 | 6027 | 1363 |
| 10-20 | R | 849 | 98 | 13 | 1000 | 22189 | 1971 |
| | U | 506 | 464 | 8 | 1000 | 5258 | 1288 |
| 20-40 | R | 823 | 134 | 8 | 1000 | 41447 | 3745 |
| | U | 436 | 535 | 7 | 1000 | 9838 | 2426 |
| 40-60 | R | 779 | 181 | 7 | 1000 | 36913 | 3463 |
| | U | 343 | 632 | 5 | 1000 | 8228 | 2176 |
| 60-80 | R | 710 | 242 | 10 | 1000 | 34235 | 3311 |
| | U | 243 | 742 | 3 | 1000 | 6451 | 1865 |
| 80-90 | R | 671 | 297 | 4 | 1000 | 14117 | 1509 |
| | U | 105 | 830 | 3 | 1000 | 3086 | 903 |
| 90-100 | R | 527 | 441 | 6 | 1000 | 10690 | 1307 |
| | U | 69 | 914 | 1 | 1000 | 2205 | 698 |
| All | R | 779 | 179 | 8 | 1000 | 185069 | 17664 |
| | U | 378 | 594 | 6 | 1000 | 41093 | 10719 |

*Source:* NSS 52nd Round, Report No. 445.

**Table 16 :** Per 1000 distribution of mothers by types of medical attention at childbirth.

| *Fractile group (All-India)* | *No. attendance* | *Govt. appointed doctor* | *Other doctor* | *Govt. appointed nurse/midwife* | *Other nurse/midwife* | *Other* | *Total** | *Numbers of mothers* | |
|---|---|---|---|---|---|---|---|---|---|
| | | | | | | | | *Estd. (00)* | *Sample* |
| 0-10 | R 482 | 28 | 16 | 71 | 168 | 205 | 1000 | 25478 | 2358 |
| | U 300 | 160 | 98 | 88 | 180 | 150 | 1000 | 6027 | 1363 |
| 10-20 | R 425 | 35 | 41 | 107 | 174 | 177 | 1000 | 22189 | 1971 |
| | U 216 | 232 | 154 | 100 | 175 | 101 | 1000 | 5258 | 1288 |
| 20-40 | R 398 | 53 | 52 | 84 | 188 | 191 | 1000 | 41447 | 3745 |
| | U 204 | 248 | 202 | 88 | 162 | 73 | 1000 | 9838 | 2426 |
| 40-60 | R 350 | 89 | 68 | 82 | 200 | 176 | 1000 | 36913 | 3463 |
| | U 104 | 264 | 296 | 85 | 187 | 44 | 1000 | 8228 | 2176 |
| 60-80 | R 278 | 108 | 129 | 82 | 219 | 145 | 1000 | 34235 | 3311 |
| | U 89 | 235 | 399 | 88 | 141 | 36 | 1000 | 6451 | 1865 |
| 80-90 | R 266 | 104 | 148 | 115 | 224 | 116 | 1000 | 14117 | 1509 |
| | U 28 | 233 | 483 | 60 | 110 | 25 | 1000 | 3086 | 903 |
| 90-100 | R 182 | 177 | 217 | 70 | 205 | 124 | 1000 | 10690 | 1307 |
| | U 25 | 124 | 721 | 19 | 78 | 12 | 1000 | 2205 | 698 |
| All | R 358 | 76 | 80 | 86 | 195 | 170 | 1000 | 185069 | 17664 |
| | U 159 | 226 | 279 | 83 | 160 | 70 | 1000 | 41093 | 10719 |

*Source:* NSS 52nd Round, Report No. 445.

employment and dignity are however overlooked (Qadeer, 1998). The economic restructuring shifts the burden of welfare from the state on to the household that inevitably means the women. Health sector reforms that promote privatisation and escalate costs of medical care, further contribute to women getting trapped in their socially constructed images. The present policies thus undermine the very basis of protection of women's health.

Further, privatisation of medical care undermines the working of all communicable disease control programmes as, in absence of adequate controls, principles of standardized treatment, data pooling, monitoring and feedbacks are sacrificed. The privatised system with its techno-centric emphasis, ignores the social roots of the problems be they of reproductive health or tuberculosis, malaria etc. Time bound, technology dependent, campaign based efforts, do not compensate for the much needed stable and functioning infrastructure that infuses confidence among the poor, promotes participation and makes monitoring and surveillance a feasible idea.

The continued strategy of adopting technocentric vertical programmes for disease control and for family welfare, are cost-ineffective and therefore wasteful. The health policy is further depleted of its strength to protect the marginalized as the state recedes from investing into welfare sector, specially public distribution system, drinking water, housing, transport and education systems. It is this overall shift from the comprehensive Primary Health Care based approach to a Primary Level Care approach that is the key to the undermining of health. Separating reproductive health from women's general health is a regressive policy and using maternity care as an excuse to push the agenda of fertility control irrespective of the safety and reliability of contraceptive technologies is simply disastrous. The Ninth Five Year Plan put contraception as its first priority under RCH (GoI, 1997) and the draft of the Tenth Five Year Plan belies all hope that the public sector health services will get the much-needed state support (GoI, 2002). Given the large chunk of population living below the poverty line or on it, and the high load of disease and under-nutrition, it is doubtful if the present RCH strategy would impact the stagnant MMRs and IMRs.

We therefore need to look back and rework policy on the basis of lessons learnt over the past decades. The need is to save and consolidate comprehensive Primary Health Care System (PHCS), which includes secondary and tertiary level care as necessary referral support for the primary level services. Without this support, services at the primary level can only be very limited and insufficient. Recourse to markets and private care may resolve some problems of the privileged but the majority of the population still remains dependent on public sector. This is so specially when people are seriously ill needing hospitalisation. While in all other civilized nations 60-100 per cent of the public sector health expenditure is contributed by the state, the Indian policy makers feel satisfied with an input of 25 per cent! They actually promotes cut backs in social sector as a whole.

If the poor and the underprivileged women have to be reach out, investing in Comprehensive Primary Health Care Services would be the first step towards meeting their health needs. Even the RCH services can succeed only as part of this system. In turn, Primary Health Care has to be a part of a social policy that emphasises inter-sectoral linkages for development—both social as well as economic.

As we saw, at present even the limited objectives of RCH are far from being met. The present health policy does little to reach out to the marginalised, and there lies the crux of its failure. As it leaves out half the population to fend for itself, it no doubt makes living difficult for the most vulnerable among them. The challenge then is not to project "average achievements" but, for each State to examine whether it has provided for its poor specially the women.

## REFERENCES

Chadha, G.K. (1999): 'Non Farm Employment in Rural Areas: How Will can Female Workers Compete?' in Papola T.S and Sharma A.N (eds): *Gender and Employment in India,* New Delhi, Vikas: 139-180.

Gupta, Jyotsna Agnihotri (2000): 'New Reproductive Technologies: Women's Health and Autonomy', New Delhi, Sage: 549-579.

Government of India (1992): *Ninth Five Year Plan, 1992-1997,* New Delhi, Planning Commission.

Government of India, Office of the Registrar General (2001): *Census of India 2001,* New Delhi, Office of the Registrar General.

Gwatkin, D.R. (2001): 'Poverty and Inequalities in Health within Developing Countries: Filling the Information Gap' in Leon D and Walt G. (ed): *Poverty, Inequality and Health: An International Perspective,* Oxford, Oxford University Press.

Illich, Ivan (1977): *Limits to Medicine,* Bombay, Rupa.

International Conference on Population and Development (1994): *ICPD Revised Draft Programme of Action,* New York, ICPD Secretariat.

International Institute for Population Sciences (1999): *National Family Health Survey-India, 1998-99,* Bombay, IIPS.

Kundu, Amitabh (1999): 'Trends and Patterns of Female Employment: A Case of Organised Informalisation' In Papola, T.S. and Sharma, A.K. (ed.) *Gender and Employment in India,* New Delhi, Vikas: 52-70.

Malobika (1993): *Girlhood in Rural Uttar Pradesh and Its Implication for Health: A Study of Two Villages of Allahabad District,* New Delhi, CSMCH (SSS), JNU, M. Phil. Dissertation.

Papola, T.S. and Sharma, A.N. (ed) (1999): *Gender and Employment in India,* New Delhi, Vikas: 104.

Rao, Mohan and Devaki Jain (2001): 'National Population Policy 2000: Re-examining Critical Issues', *Economic and Political Weekly,* Vol. 36, No., 16, April 21:1299-1302.

Richter, Judith (1993): *Vaccination Against Pregnancy: Miracle or Menace?* Amsterdam, Health Action International.

Sagar, Alpana (2001): 'The Reproductive Health Package: A Chimera for Women's Health' in Qadeer, Imrana, Sen Kasturi and K.R. Nayar (ed): *Public Health and the Poverty of Reforms: The South Asian Predicament,* New Delhi, Sage: 504-523.

Sathyamala, C. (2001): *An Epidemiological Review of the Injectable, Contraceptive Depo-Provera,* Pune, Medico Friends Circle.

Sen, Abhijit (1996): 'Economic Reform, Employment and Poverty: Trends and Options', *Economic and Political Weekly,* Vol. 31, Nos. 35-37, 2459-2578.

Sen, Gita, Asha George and Pirosk Ostlin (ed) (2002): *Engendering International Health: The Challenge of Equity,* London, MIT Press.

Soman, Krishna (1992): *An Exploratory Study of Social Dynamics of Women's Health in Adityapur Village of Birbhum District,* New Delhi, CSMCH (SSS), JNU, M. Phil Dissertation.

Srivastava, Nisha (1999): 'Striving for a Toe-hold: Women in the Organized Sector' in Papola, T.S. and Sharma A.N. (ed.): *Gender and Employment in India,* New Delhi, Vikas: 181-205.

Sundaram, K. (2001): 'Employment and Policy', *Economic and Political Weekly* August 7-14, 2001: 3039-3049.

Qadeer, Imrana (1998): 'Reproductive Health: A Public Health Perspective', *Economic and Political Weekly,* Vol. 33, October 10: 2675-2684.

Qadeer, Imrana (2001): 'Public Health Perspective for Reproductive Health of Women', *Vikalp-Alternatives,* Vol. 9, Nos. 1-2: 61-72.

# 2

# ABOUT THE REPRODUCTIVE AND CHILD HEALTH PROGRAMME

*Pradeep Padwal*

The Reproductive and Child Health Programme introduced by the Government of India since 1995 aims at addressing the health needs of women from womb to tomb. The programme includes the early registration of pregnancy, regular antenatal check-up, T. T. immunisation, prevention and treatment of anaemia in expectant mothers, early identification of high risk cases, promotion of institutional deliveries, essential new-born and post-natal care, promotion of exclusive breast feeding, growth monitoring and effective immunisation of infants, vitamin A supplementation, supplementary nutrition advice with attention to the girl child, treatment and referral services for management of severe mal-nutrition, diarrhoeal diseases and ARI to minimise childhood diseases to safeguard maternal and child health and to minimize MMR and IMR. The programme also includes the strict implementation of the PNDT Act which will not only curb the female foeticide practices but also ensure a healthy male : female ratio.

The programme aims at the promotion of adolescent health and sexuality education to ensure responsible parenthood and avoid unplanned and unwanted pregnancies as well as unsafe abortions, reduce the prevalence of STDs and HIV/AIDS. The programme will provide couples with sound knowledge of spacing and terminal methods like sterilizations.

he RCH programme will encourage regular health check-ups or early detection of breast cancer, cervical cancer and other ilments coupled with advice on post-menopausal and age elated health problems.

## Paradigm Shift

he 1994 ICPD established an international consensus on a ew approach to policies to achieve population stabilisation. his highlighted that fertility reduction concerns should be ddressed at the level of broad social policy and should nclude also the reduction of gender discrimination in ducation, health care and work. It was felt that reproductive ealth programmes should focus on the needs of actual and otential clients, not only for limiting births but for healthy xuality and child bearing. In India, the implications of the productive health approach implied a shift in the focus from e use of family planning as a tool intended essentially for opulation stabilisation to using family planning as one among constellation of intervention that would enable women and en to achieve their personal reproductive goals without ing subjected to the additional burdens of disease and death sociated with their reproduction. Such a shift in emphasis ould be more likely to address the needs of women who are risk of having unwanted births, and in so doing assist the untry to accelerate fertility decline. Reproductive health terventions would enable clients to make informed choices, receive counselling and education for responsible and healthy xual behaviour, to access user-friendly services for preventing wanted pregnancy and safe abortion, maternity care and ild survival; and management of reproductive tract infections TIs). The Government of India (GoI) has increasingly dorsed these views and its country statement strongly reflects e principles of ICPD's Programme of Action.

Over the years of implementation of the Family Welfare ogramme in India, it was felt that people have not responded the services provided enthusiastically due to many reasons: . The programme does not address completely the needs of omen and children: the programme is not in tune with the plementation needs of the health workers: workload of the programme has not been set with consideration to the loca demographic and health needs of the population etc. In respons to these needs the government has now reoriented the famil welfare programme to provide an integrated package o services. The new RCH programme aims to improve th monthly coverage, effectiveness and access of services. Th programme has adopted an entirely new approach and th components of paradigm shift in the programme are briefl indicated below:

*Target Free Programme from April 1996*

In April 1996, Government of India took a landmark decisio to withdraw the system of estimating workload as well a monitoring the programme based on centrally determine method, that is, the contraceptive target system. Instead adopted a Community Need Assessment (CNA) based bottor up approach where self-estimated goals/workload were use by the health workers.

*Decentralised Participatory Planning*

Planning actually begins at the grass root level/village lev with members of Panchayat and Mahila Swasthya Sangh an other persons closely interacting with the ANM and ma health worker for deciding about the actual requirement various family welfare services. This improves the sustainabili of the programme by having sense of involvement and th community owning the programme thereby increasir utilisation of services as well as by ensuring a sense responsibility and accountability among the workers.

The plans are prepared for sub-centres which a aggregated to make the PHC plans which in turn ge aggregated to form the district plan.

*Integrated RCH Package*

Integrated RCH package includes essential RCH package whi gives basic minimum model framework of RCH services different levels in the district *viz.* CHC, PHC, FRU and distr hospital. The essential components are:

- Prevention and management of unwanted pregnancy.
- Maternal care including antenatal, intranatal and post-natal services.
- Child survival services including new born care.
- Management of RTI/STI.

*State/District Specific RCH Strategy*

Considering the variations in regard to various parameters/ indicators states and districts area specific approach has been worked out separately for different groups of states and districts. States and districts classified based on parameters like CPR, TFR, female literacy level, percentage women registered for ANC, percentage of hospital delivery, percentage delivered by untrained birth attendant etc. Additional inputs are provided to poor performing states and districts.

*Greater Emphasis on Quality*

Provision of good quality care is the crux of the RCH programme. Good quality care ensures client satisfaction which is one of the major goals of the programme. This in turn would increase the service utilisation. Therefore provision of good quality care by health personnel would determine the success of the programme.

In service training of health personnel with due focus on practical skills is a major input for improving quality of care. Need has also been felt for shift from vertical training structure with training in different components of care at different locations and different times to a comprehensive RCH training package which would include clinical components as well as managerial and communication components.

*Comprehensive Integrated Raining with District as the Coordinator*

An important feature of the training in future will be the field functionaries and the Anganwadi workers as well as functionaries from other development sectors. Planning and management of training programme would be th responsibility of the district Central and State Government will support the district in training of trainers and productio of training materials.

*Increase Involvement of NGOs and Private Sector*

Service providers from NGO and private sector are involve in the delivery of services as well as in providing training anc for IEC, Social marketing of contraceptives and RCH product is another area of involvement.

*Area Specific IEC Campaigns*

While there is attempt to evolve national IEC strategy for RCH emphasis is placed on development of local areas specific communication strategies to create more demand for RCH services and to promote informed decision-making for use of services. Thus, health personnel are trained in IEC skills to motivate people for use of right kind of meeting their needs. Special emphasis is also placed of IPC and use of local traditional media for increasing acceptance and impact.

*Change in Financing Mechanism*

Direct financing of states through Standing Committee for Voluntary Action (SCOVA) with the objectives of avoiding delays in implementation due to budgetary constraints have been started.

*Change in Procurement Practices*

A National Procurement Support Agency (NPSA) has been hired to enable smooth supply of goods and services to ensure transparency in procurement practices. Similar agencies are being set-up in states also.

*Management Information System*

The CNA approach is participatory planning and monitoring

with involvement of stake holders (women and men). The reporting system including items reported has undergone change and the indicators developed from the reports are also changed.

*Introduction of Quality and Impact Indicators*

Alternative quality and impact indicators are replacing the method specific contraceptive and other quantitative targets for monitoring programme. Good quality care assessed through process indicators prompt service, increasing accessibility etc. are being used.

*Independent/Rapid Evaluation*

The system of monitoring and evaluation has undergone changes. It is participatory involving different stake holders and focus is on quality. Evaluation by PRCs and other independent teams has been introduced through household and health facility surveys which provide data regularly for enabling corrective actions as and when needed. Quality of services based on clients health seeking behaviour will also be monitored/evaluated.

*Gender Concerns*

All efforts have been made to make the programme as gender-sensitive as possible. Women's groups are involved in planning and monitoring.

*Increased Male Participation in the Programme*

Need for increased male participation in the RCH programme has been given considerable importance. More responsibility in child rearing by males, increase acceptance of male contraception informed decision-making for service use jointly by males and females, male participation in RCH service provision etc. are important.

*Multi-sectoral Participation in Health and Nutrition Services*

Convergence with other sectors for success of the programme particularly for nutrition has been given due consideration. Awareness generation training programmes are planned for functionaries from all developmental sectors.

*Involvement of Panchayati Raj System*

Panchayati Raj System is expected to play a significant role in planning for RCH services particularly for identification of the needs of local population for RCH services. The system is also to play a role in the implementation, particularly financial support and transport for referral of women to hospitals for deliveries. For evaluation of the programme the Panchayat system extends supports in assessing the client satisfaction. Therefore special efforts to produce RCH awareness training to Panchayat members is envisaged.

*RCH Services for Special Population Groups*

Certain vulnerable segments population like tribal population, urban slum deliveries, adolescents who have prominent specific service needs for RCH need to be addressed through specially designed additional programmes/projects.

*Addition or Special Focus on Certain Service Components*

Two service components have been added to essential RCH package *viz.* Prevention and management of RTI and STDs. Under comprehensive RCH Programme care of gynaecological morbidity as well as infertility management screening and management of cancers are also added special focus is also given on provision of safe abortion services.

*Adolescent Health and Forty Plus Care*

Adolescent health and forty plus care are two new dimensions well focused under the RCH package services to address the specific problems of adolescents and elderly group of people.

## List of 50 Comprehensive RCH Services

**I. Maternal and Child Health**

1. Early registration of pregnancy
2. Antenatal check up.
3. TT immunisation.
4. Prevention and treatment of Anemia in mothers.
5. Early identification of high risk cases.
6. Deliveries by trained personnel.
7. Promiton of institutional deliveries.
8. Essential new-born care.
9. Post-natal care.
10. Exclusive breast feeding and weaning.
11. Growth monitoring.
12. Immunisation (including Pulse Polio and MMR)
13. Rubella immunisation.
14. Vitamin A prophylaxis.
15. Prevention and treatment of Anemia in children.

**II. Nutrition**

16. Supplementary nutrition and nutrition advice with attention to the girl child.
17. Treatment of severely malnourished children.

**III. Management of Childhood Diseases**

18. Appropriate management of diarrhoea.
19. Appropriate management of ARI.

**IV. Referral Services**

20. Management of obstetrical emergencies.
21. Paediatric referral services.

**V. Fertility**

22. Spacing and terminal methods.
23. Safe abortion.
24. Advice and treatment to sterility cases.

**VI. Population and Sexuality Education**

25. Population and its effects.
26. Physical and psychological changes during early adolescence.

27. Sex education.
28. adolescent health.
29. Human sexuality.
30. Family life education.
31. Responsible parenthood.
32. Pre-marriage counselling.

**VII. Reproductive Tract and Sexually Transmitted Infections**

33. RTI
34. STD
35. AIDS

**VIII. Gender Issues**

36. Male responsibility and participation.
37. Gender equality.
38. Equality and empowerment of women.

**IX. Education**

39. Non-formal education.
40. Primary education with emphasis on education of the girl child.
41. School health examination
42. Personal hygiene.
43. Secondary education.
44. Vocational training especially for girls.

**X. Forty Plus Care**

45. Regular health check-up after 40 years of age.
46. Diagnosis and treatment of breast cancer.
47. Diagnosis and treatment of cervical cancer.
48. Diagnosis and treatment of cancers at other sites.
49. Diagnosis and treatment of other gynaecological and health problems.
50. Old age problems.

*Source :* Reproductive and Child Health Programme: A Comprehensive Package of RCH Services, Dr. G. A. Panse, Pune 1999, V.R Publications and Publications of National Institute of Health and Family Welfare.

# 3

# MEETING WOMEN'S HEALTH NEEDS

## Dynamics of State Policy and Programme

*Shaila Desouza*

Right up to the 1990s, the prime agenda of India's family health and welfare programme was to increase the number of women who were sterilized and to motivate 'eligible' women, that is women in the reproductive age group of 15-45 years, to use family planning methods. Neglecting other issues concerning family health, the programme focused chiefly on population control.

In 1994 the International Conference on Population and Development (ICPD) held in Cairo, articulated the need for a global change in this limited understanding of health and well-being. The deliberations at this conference were undoubtedly influenced by the demands of the women's movement for a more holistic approach to health. Much was also drawn from feminist visions of 'empowerment', which highlighted the importance of women's rights including the right of women to control 'her' own body. A total of 179 countries ratified the resolutions of the ICPD of which, India was one. These resolutions thus facilitated a shift in the 'stated' focus of health policy from population control to reproductive health and rights. However in the actual health service delivery the experience was no different as we will see through this paper.

The new Reproductive and Child Health programme was introduced all over the country in 1995. Literature on this programme articulates that, it aims at a decentralised and more participatory planning process, a target free approach to health care, an emphasis on provision of quality services and that it places a premium on meeting women's health needs through the Community Needs Assessment approach. This programme at first glance seemed to be pro-women but when examined more closely what is more apparent is the lack of a clear design for proper implementation. There is also no assured budgetary provision to make the dream of meeting community needs possible. Examining the programme as it is being implemented today one is unfortunately forced to believe that this is just 'old wine in a new bottle'.

## The Experience of Goa in the Early 1990s

### *The Target was then Numbers*

The author of this paper was involved from late 1980's to early 1990s in projects of the Indian Council for Medical Research (ICMR) and the Integrated Child Development Scheme (ICDS) based in rural Goa, which were conducted through the Human Reproduction Research Centre, attached to the Goa Medical College. The following is based on some of these experiences.

The work in the Human Reproduction Research Centre (HRRC) in Goa began in mid 1980. At that time in Goa an aggressive contraceptive target system was in place with a monetary incentive and a disincentive scheme too. The efforts of the State Health Department were to reduce fertility as quickly as possible. The highest target and incentive was available for sterilization, followed by IUD. In fact the Provedoria, which was then under the Department of Social Welfare and which was exclusive to the State of Goa gave additional monetary incentives making sterilization in Goa almost a profitable business. According to the Directorate of Health Services, Goa, at that time, the State Health Department gave Rs. 100 and the Provedoria Rs. 220 for each sterilization. Contraceptive targets or rather the number of persons in the area who were to be enrolled as contraceptive users were set at the state level and delegated downwards making it the responsibility of the auxiliary nurse midwives (ANM's) to find 'contraceptive acceptors'. Sometimes the assigned targets were much higher than what was realistically possible. In some areas there were not sufficient 'eligible' women who wanted to practice contraception, specifically the contraception as was being offered by the Primary Health Care programme of the government. Therefore the job of the ANM's was not an easy one. They had to know their area well by making frequent home visits. They were also expected to maintain an updated 'eligible couples register', motivate persons who also might have been opposed to contraceptive technology and preferred natural methods. They also had sometimes to scout out for persons outside their 'catchment' area. Apart from that the ANM's were also required to hold weekly clinics for immunisation, antenatal check-ups, distribution of condoms and oral contraceptive pills, treatment of minor illnesses and sometimes had even to attend to deliveries. These health functionaries were therefore so overworked with no real compensation for their efforts. Women and child health care in reality were neglected, as there was no concern given to other health concerns of the public.

The ANM's aspired for better postings as rewards for their achievement of targets and feared transfers to undesirable work areas for not fulfilling their assigned targets. Some health functionaries who feared this sort of 'punishment' employed various tactics to meet the targets. The strategies adopted include the trading and procuring of 'sterilization candidates' from areas outside their own. Health workers who were unable to meet their targets would often try to get cases from other PHC areas and sometimes even from outside the state. Another strategy adopted to meet the target was the inclusion of women who were not on their eligible couple's list like widows, women who had reached menopause or whose husbands had already undergone a vasectomy.

Health workers would pay special attention to women in their area who fitted the profile of a prospective candidate for sterilization. Like for example women who were expecting their second child. In fact there were cases when a woman going in for her second delivery would be accompanied by the health worker to the hospital. This was done with a hope that she was a prospective sterilization candidate it was not done with a concern for that woman's health. Women with two or more children were literally hounded to accept contraception. Motivation was aggressive and sometimes relentless and therefore the community always suspected the intention of any health worker who happened to visit the area.

An important point of criticism of this programme was that there was little or no attention given to after care or follow up of these users. Women in the community became mere numerical figures and objects for use rather than persons that had to be served by the health department.

At this juncture I would like to discuss the practice at that time of conducting sterilization camps.

### *Camps to Increase Numbers*

The race to meet targets was so fierce that numbers had to be increased at any cost. The sterilization camps were testimony to this fact. Women were sterilized in large numbers in these camps. In Goa these camps were most often conducted by doctors from outside the State and were conducted in PHC premises.

The following is the narration of experiences in one such camp that the author observed along with a team from the HRRC. On the 28th October, 1988, we got the opportunity to observe a laparascopic camp in a Primary Health Centre in Goa (SAAD, 1994). 129 women were 'ligated' that day by one doctor, assisted by his wife who was the anesthetist. The doctor couple completed all 129 operations before lunch. The doctors boasted about the speed with which they were able to work but no mention was made of precision and care. The infrastructure in the hospital itself did not allow for human operative and post-operative care to be given to more than about 30 to 40 cases (at a generous estimate). When the operations began, pre-medication was given to the patients but the first 30 odd cases were operated too soon after medication and were not completely sedated and were therefore very anxious. This was worsened as the doors of the operation theatre were kept open and those waiting in turn outside could clearly see and hear the screams and shouts of the patients being operated before them. No operation gowns were given to the patients, most of who were in *'sarees'* and were simply made to strip into their underskirts and *'cholis'*. They were, needless to say, very embarrassed and self-conscious.

Each operation took not more than 3 to 4 minutes. Four laparascopes were used in rotation for all the operations giving a maximum of 9-12 minutes for each instrument to be sterilized before it was re-used. In the operation theatre, make shift operating tables were set up with benches, tables and stools. The benches were kept with a head-low tilt. As there were no stirrups to hold the patients from sliding down, each patient had to hold herself up with her legs hanging free over the edge of the table. Several patients complained of severe calf muscle cramps post-operatively, which might have been caused by this position during the operation.

The patients were made to walk out of the operation theatre immediately after the operation. One woman fainted and although there was a stretcher available, she was just lifted out by three male attendants and taken to the post-operative room.

The post-operative room was one long dormitory, with mattresses lined on the floor. Patients were crowded side by side in the room which, was not properly ventilated. It was hot and stuffy with all the windows shut and only one fan in working condition. Most of the patients in the room were partially sedated though some were restless and were trying to sit up. Some were vomiting on the sheets or even on each other as there were insufficient vomit bowls and staff to attend to the patients needs. The common complaints were severe colic and as mentioned before calf muscle pain.

There was no doctor available in the post-operative room and ANM's present hesitated to call doctors. Only some patients had their relatives or ANMs with them. Several looked on helplessly. When we interviewed the women we learnt that several had not told their husbands about the operation. Several had in fact been advised by the ANMs, especially those that suspected a refusal of permission from their spouses, that there would be no stitches required and that only a small incision would be made which could go undetected by one's spouse too. The marketing strategy was that the patient could go home in a day. After 3 to 4 hours of post-operative stay the patients were transported home in ambulances or made their own way home. Our interview with the motivators revealed that they did not inform patients about the after effects of the operation least it discourage patients who already had a fear of such procedures. Of course cash rewards for those undergoing the treatment was used as the bait.

At the camps that were witnessed, the number of patients was always more than was possible for the hospital facilities to ensure quality care or any follow up for.

What needs to be highlighted is the fact that although patients suffered pain, embarrassment and dissatisfaction, never once was any form of protest raised about the manner in which they were being treated. The women were silent acceptors of these procedures. Doctors were almost held as gods. They were probably unaware of what they could have demanded for, and that they deserved better treatment that was not only their right but something that could have easily been made possible. The rest of the public were little aware of what was happening and are still probably unaware of these aspects of the health programme. Fortunately these camps have been discontinued. When the camps were discontinued there were no explanations given to the public or even health functionaries for that matter for this discontinuance and therefore no guarantee that it will not be reintroduced.

This experience was shared by projects that were being conducted elsewhere in India too (Karkal, 1993; Verma, *et al.*, 1999; Murthy, 2002 etc.). According to the National Family Health Survey (1998-99) ¾ of the population that are considered as 'contraceptive users' in India have been sterilized. The monetary incentive for sterilization plays no small role in this. However the NFHS also revealed that most women who chose sterilization were those who already had an average of 4 children. Therefore it would not be wrong to state that the policy failure and the one of the reasons for a marginal change in the policy today was that the primary aim of controlling population by limiting child birth through sterilization failed, and second, this policy is a drain on the finances of the state due to the incentive structure provided for sterilization. One however cannot help worrying what the response of the government will be if an outside agency would offer to bear the financial cost of such a programme. According to the Directorate of Health Services, Goa, the incentive money today is Rs. 100 for the acceptor, diet Rs. 30, transport Rs. 15, drugs and dressings Rs. 25, and miscellaneous Rs. 30. Of this the patient can only claim the first two *i.e.* Rs. 100 plus 30 for diet. The rest is claimed by the hospital.

The aggressive contraceptive target system was a violation of women's health rights as it focused little or no attention on real health needs of the women in the community. The women had no rights to choose whether they wanted or not to use a particular contraceptive device, they had no right to quality services and no right to an informed consent. When a monetary incentive for a medical procedure exists, the consent given cannot be considered 'voluntary' especially in a Third World countries where large scale poverty exists and the incentive money can blind reason. The author's experience with the project of the HRRC was that although consent forms were signed by the patients rarely were these voluntary and informed consents. The same is true for the contraceptive trials that are being conducted even today in the name of research. The public is not informed of the trials that are being conducted through the state hospitals and neither is the literature on the trial drugs or contraceptive methods made available to the general public. Then, when the trials are discontinued there is no follow up commitment to patients registered in the trials and neither is the public informed of the reasons for the discontinuation of the trial. There was and still is little transparency and accountability to the public in these so-called research projects despite the use of public funds. Besides if data generated in the state is to be credible it should also be made accessible to the public.

## Aggressive Marketing and Poor Local Response in Goa

Despite the aggressive marketing strategies like media

promotion, targets, financial incentives and disincentives that were being used to promote contraceptive use, the present response of the Goan community to modern contraceptive technology is very poor (according to National Family Health Survey data). Reasons for this could be attributed to several things, including poor quality of care and the experience of side effects.

In the state of Goa, which has the second highest literacy rate in the country, knowledge of family planning is universal (99%) according to NFHS-1 (1991-92) and NFHS-2 (1998-99) both in the rural areas as well as the urban areas and sterilization is better known than spacing methods. Yet the current contraceptive prevalence of currently married women is 48 per cent, which is the same as the national average. Of the total contraceptive prevalence female sterilization accounts for 59 per cent (NFHS-2)

NFHS data has also revealed that the use of sterilization decreases as the level of education increases. The rate of sterilization among illiterate women was 48 per cent (NFHS-2) and the rate of sterilization among literate women was only 12 per cent (NFHS-2).

Sterilization use has also shown to decline as the standard of living increases. The sterilization use among women from households with a low standard of living was 42 per cent (NFHS-2) and that among women from house holds with a high standard of living was only 19 per cent.

It may be pertinent to note that the current use of modern contraceptive methods have declined from 38 per cent (NFHS-1) to 34 per cent (NFHS-2) and it is interesting to note that the use of modern methods is higher among the rural women than the urban women.

On the other hand, the use of traditional methods has increased from 10 per cent (NFHS-1) to 12 per cent (NFHS-2) And surprising to note that the use of traditional methods by urban women is three times as high as that of the rural women. The use of traditional methods also increases sharply with household standard of living.

The rates of use of modern contraception and traditional methods by illiterate women is

| | 1991-92 | 1998-99 |
|---|---|---|
| Modern methods | 43% | 53% |
| Traditional methods | 4% | 3% |

while that among with at least high school education is

| | 1991-92 | 1998-99 |
|---|---|---|
| Modern methods | 29% | 40% |
| Traditional methods | 21% | 17% |

According to the NFHS 1 and 2, the practice of contraception is strongly related to the level of education of the women. The current use of 'modern' methods is lower among women with high school education and above, than among illiterate women, although the average family size among those with education is less than that of those who are illiterate.

The public sector consisting of government, municipal hospitals, primary health centres and other government health institutions, supplies three-fourths of all modern methods used in Goa.

Interestingly however, despite this low contraceptive acceptance or use in Goa, the fertility rate in the state is low. It has attained a below replacement level with a TFR of 1.9 children per woman (NFHS-1) and 1.77 children per woman (NFHS-2) as against the national average of 2.9 children per woman. Unwanted fertility in Goa is also low. It must be noted that in Goa the age at marriage is also high, which is approximately 25 years.

My question is, what happens if the fertility rate in the state should increase. Will the old policy be re-started? Why isn't the public informed about these policy decisions and explanations given for changes? Should the public not be made aware of what affects them the most?

## Shift in Policy

The focus of the health programme today following the ICPD conference in 1994 was reproductive and child health and more importantly the acknowledgment of the importance of a responding to community needs which is now referred to as

RCH and CNA (Community Needs Assessment). The CNA programme has only general guidelines and leaves the finer details to be worked out by each state according to what is possible for each state to implement. The health workers to be more specific the paramedical workers are given the responsibility to conduct CNA's and then consult with medical officers when making the work plan for implementation.

'Quality services'are the catch-words for the RCH program. According to the literature on this programme, the health workers are required to set targets for themselves as performance goals. Contraceptive use however does not cease to be a programmatic goal. The new programme at a cursory glance at the existing literature circulated by the Ministry for Health and Family Welfare utters a language that seems to be similar to the demands of the feminist movement. However when studied more closely, and when one assesses the field implementation of the programme, one distressingly learns that it 'is' merely old wine in a new bottle. This sometimes is more frightening than the earlier programme. It almost silences all forms of protest (the little that may exists) with it's pro-women appearance but in reality sustains all the elements of the previous programme. This programme in several ways takes the wind out of feminist protests while in reality remains largely unchanged.

The RCH and CNA programme yet lacks clarity regarding strategies to meet the programme's objectives. Much of the success of the programme has been stated to rely on the paramedical functionaries, meaning the Auxiliary Nurse Midwives and the Basic Health Workers who in the hierarchy of the health functionaries are almost at the bottom end. The RCH programme lists out the tasks that have to be accomplished with a rather warped load on the ANMs and BHWs while the more trained professionals escape without any such pressure. Of the 50 services listed out as the services to be implemented through the RCH programme (Panse, 1999), 26 services are to be undertaken only by the paramedical staff (ANMs and BHWs) and in fact there are 37 services that are their responsibilities. Besides if one looks at the types of services that are chalked out as responsibilities of the para-medicals, all the preventive services, counselling, health education and promotive services are their responsibility. With this increased number of services offered there is obviously a tremendous increase in work load as there has not been an increase in the staff structure in the sub-centres nor has there been any increase in budgetary allocation. The new programme does not really do away with the target system nor the monetary incentive system. The change here is that the para-medical staff set performance goals for themselves after consultation at the PHC and District levels and these goals are set based on data they collect in their survey's to update the Family Register. Informal interviews with health functionaries reveal that senior health officials suspect the ANM's and BHW's of intentionally underreporting the community needs so that they can set lower performance goals for themselves. Some para-medical staff feel that the hierarchies have not changed but the power dynamics have taken a new form.

The literature on the Community Needs Assessment commits to meeting community needs through the programme. However the existing implementation of CNA however is that the para-medical staff update the Family Register in which they record family planning status, vaccination status, a few illness such as TB, leprosy, STD/RTI's, blindness/cataract, vector borne diseases, drinking water sources and physical handicaps. This data from the survey to update the Family Register then becomes the assessment of community needs. There is no real involvement of the community in identifying actual needs. There is little or no involvement of local representatives of the community like NGO's, women's groups, panchayats etc., in problem identification, planning and implementation. There is no empowerment project for the community to be able to identify their health needs, make demands for their requirements and be assured of their demands being adequately met.

If one were to look at existing data on the issues concerning women's health one would clearly be able to state that not all the issues listed in the Family Register are the most immediate concerns of women in Goa.

Some Worrying Figures from the NFHS-2 are :

| | |
|---|---|
| Women involved in decisions about their own health care | 62% |

| | |
|---|---|
| Anemia (including moderate +severe) among women is | 36.4% |
| Anemia among children (6 months to 3 years) is | 53.4% |
| Children chronically undernourished (stunted) | 18.1% |
| Children acutely undernourished (wasted) | 13.1% |
| Children underweight | 28.6% |
| Total children undernourished and at risk | 59.8% |

If this is the position of infants and children, how much worse would be that of women?

The NFHS-2 revealed that 27.1 per cent of the pregnant women have low body mass index and this is during the period when women are comparatively better fed.

With regards to other NFHS-2 data which could be indicators of health status, only 63.6 per cent households are within 15 mins. walking distance from safe water supply and this includes pipes, hand-pumps, covered wells etc. Only 62 per cent households have piped drinking water. Only 38 per cent households have flush toilets and 41 per cent households have no toilet at all.

These are just some indicators of issues that might be revealed from the existing data sources. The program to be successful has to take the community into confidence and involve actively at all levels of the programme, NGO's, women's groups, leaders in the community including also the panchayats etc.

The situation in Goa today is that at the village level in people's eyes, little has changed. The changes if any in the programme have not been noticed. The public does not see any real change in quality of services after the CNA/RCH programme and most people have not even heard about the decentralized planning or about the removal of targets/ incentives. At present there are financial constraints and pressure on the already overworked female para-medical staff.

## Concluding Comments

I end here with a few anxieties about the health policy and

programme. Methods of community assessment are important. If a Family Register is used with only yes and no responses asked for, with only specific health issues being enquired about, the questions asked may not reflect the real health needs of the community. For example the questions could only be focused on reproductive health and not touch upon issues like malnutrition, alcoholism, mental health, violence etc. However, with the present budgetary allocation would the health care system realistically be able to meet women's health needs? Issues that continue to be unclear are the management of the programme. The planning seems to be decentralized but there is no indication of a decentralized implementation.

An important aspect in assessing community health needs is reaching a common understanding of the term 'health'. This continues to be ambiguous, particularly with reference to women's health. The ambiguity arises from the divergent understanding of the needs for the well-being of the human body even for example between the modern clinic-based western science and traditional health practices (Desouza, 2000). This has been completely ignored by state health policy. What I am saying here is that in our society there may be varied and unique perceptions of well-being and therefore disease or ill health. The acceptance and perpetuation of one or the other system is dependent on state policy and community's own experience (tradition and affordability) of either system. It is time that the state initiates some process by which these systems can not only be understood but also incorporated into main stream health care.

Finally, since data in NFHS 1 and 2 has pointed out that in Goa the response to modern contraception is low, it is possible that the outcome of the Community Needs Assessment could also reveal that the women's need for contraception is far lower than the government expectation. With population control not completely off the agenda, how would the government respond. Accountability to the public in terms of policy and changes therein should be the state's responsibility to its citizens.

## REFERENCES

Desouza, Shaila (2000): 'Health Practices and People's Identity: Re-Locating Identity', Lusotopie 2000 : *Enjeux Contemporains Dans Les Espaces Lusophones,* Lusophonies asiatiques, Asiatiques en lusophonies, Volume publie avec les concours du CNRS (Paris) et de la Comissao nacional para as Comemoracoes dos Descobrimentos portugueses (Lisbonne), Pasis Karthala: 764, ISBN : 2-84586-146-X.

Government of India, Department of Family Welfare, Ministry of Health and Family Welfare (1997): *Reproductive and Child Health Programme: Schemes for Implementation.*

Government of India, Department of Family Welfare, Ministry of Health and Family Welfare (1998): *Manual on Community Needs Assessment Approach in Family Welfare Programme.*

International Institute for Population Sciences, Bombay (1995): *National Family Health Survey: MCH and Family Planning: India 1992-1993.*

International Institute for Population Sciences, Bombay and Population Research Centre, J.S.S Institute of Economic Research, Dharwad, Karnataka (1995): *National Family Health Survey: MCH and Family Planning: Goa 1992-1993.*

International Institute for Population Sciences, Mumbai and Measure DHS+, ORC Macro, Calverton, Maryland, USA (March 2002): *National Family Health Survey - 2: Goa 1998-1999.*

Karkal, Malini (1993): 'Population Control and International Politics', Paper presented at the VIth National Conference of the Indian Association for Women's Studies, Mysore.

Murthy, Nirmala *et al.* (2002): 'Dismantling India's Contraception Target System', in Haberland, Nicole and Diana Measham (eds), *Responding to Cairo: Case Studies of Changing Practice in Reproductive Health and Family Planning,* New York: Population Council: 25 -57.

Panse, G.A. (1999): *Reproductive and Child Health Programme: A Comprehensive Package of 50 Services to be Provided over 12 Phases,* Pune, V.R Publications.

SAAD (1994): Newsletter of Bailancho Saad, Vol. I No.3 dated 11.07.94, page 7.

Verma, Ravi K. and T.K. Roy (1999): 'Assessing the Quality of Family Planning Service Providers in Four Indian States' in Koenig M. A. and M.E. Khan (eds), *Improving Quality of Care in India's Family Welfare Programme: The Challenge Ahead.* New York: Population Council: 169-182.

Visaria, Leela (1999): 'The Quality of Reproductive Health Care in Gujarat: Perspectives of Female Health Workers and their Clients' in Koenig M.A. and M.E. Khan (eds), *Improving Quality of Care in India's Family Welfare Programme: The Challenge Ahead.* New York: Population Council: 143-168.

# MENTAL HEALTH ISSUES

# 4

# INVISIBLE WOMEN

## Issues in the Care and Reintegration of Women with Severe Mental Illness

*Prabha S. Chandra*

Women with severe mental illness (schizophrenia, bipolar affective disorders and chronic depression ) form a sizeable part of the population. Unfortunately, a large majority of these women do not come into contact with services and facilities other than those for acute psychiatric care. Available services for rehabilitation and after care are biased towards men and have not focused on the special needs of women patients. This causes major obstacles in reintegrating mentally ill women back into society. Women with chronic mental illness usually have problems in social skills, negotiation,communication and judgement, that may impair marital relationships, affect parenting and child rearing and negatively influence family relationships. This leads to further stigma and discrimination and over time women with severe mental illness become invisible to society. They are not considered as contributing members of society, have no roles in families and cannot advocate for themselves. In addition, living in the fringes of families and society, they are often subject to abuse, psychological, physical and sexual-abuse that is not evident or reported. Not having voices to speak for themselves and few caregivers and health professionals as their advocates, women with SMI become truly invisible and their needs remain unmet.

Mental illnesses affect women and men differently—some disorders are more common in women, and some express themselves with different symptoms. Scientists are only now beginning to tease apart the contribution of various biological and psychosocial factors to mental health and mental illness in both women and men. In addition, researchers are currently studying the special problems of treatment for serious mental illness during pregnancy and the post-partum period. Research on women's health has grown substantially in the last 20 years. Today's studies are helping to clarify the risk and protective factors for mental disorders in women and to improve women's mental health treatment outcome.

During recent years, there has been an increase in the interest paid to gender differences in psychiatry, possibly as a result of the political processes that have been initiated by women themselves (Bennet, 1993). While the information available is as yet limited, it is already evident that major gender differences exist in the prevalence, clinical manifestations, response to treatment, and course of all major psychiatric disorders and hence the approaches to women and men with severe mental illness need to consider these specific needs.

In many matters related to women and chronic mental illness, serious lacunae in knowledge exist; for example, when new psychotropic drugs are released, little information is available about gender-specific effects of these drugs, and their impact on menstruation, pregnancy, and lactation (Markata *et al.*, 1993). Furthermore, psychosocial programmes rarely keep issues specific to women on their agenda; most rehabilitation settings have common programmes for men and women. Psychopharmacological and psychosocial issues are both of concern because it is becoming increasingly apparent that female psychiatric patients require a different approach to management (Chandra and Vijaylakshmi, 2000).

The scope of this paper, therefore, is to highlight aspects of importance in the field of chronic mental illness in women; disorders considered are depression, bipolar disorder, and schizophrenia.

Four important areas emerge when discussing the specific needs of women with severe mental illness in the community.

(a) Marriage, pregnancy and child rearing.
(b) Major mental illness and gynaecological care.
(c) Major mental illness and sexuality.
(d) Violence in mentally ill women.

**Practical Issues Related to Pregnancy**

In women with chronic mental illness, as in other stigmatized and marginalized groups, the desire to become pregnant may be intensified because child-bearing is one source of self-esteem that can be pursued despite multiple losses in the role functioning as a consequence of the illness. However, pregnancy poses several problems to the mentally ill woman. Certain of these problems are considered in the sections that follow.

*Diagnosis of Pregnancy*

The diagnosis of pregnancy may be difficult as mentally ill women are poor self-observers or may deny pregnancy. Caregivers ( Family and Health Professionals) should therefore keep records of patients' contraceptive practices and menstrual cycles. Caregivers should also maintain a high level of alertness for possible pregnancy, and should ask for pregnancy tests whenever there is a suspicion that a patient may be pregnant.

*Prenatal Concerns*

Women with chronic mental illness are more likely to have unwanted pregnancies, and more likely to be older, unemployed, and homeless (Miller *et al.*, 1992). Poor prenatal care is consequently common. Risk for pregnancy-related complications therefore increases, and this risk is compounded by the increased prevalence of substance abuse, poverty, and poor nutrition in such patients (Rudolph *et al.*, 1990).

Psychotic denial of a confirmed pregnancy is rare but

potentially dangerous; it is associated with a diagnosis of schizophrenia, a history of loss of custody of children, and a fear of future loss of custody (Miller, 1990). Potential risks involved in the denial of pregnancy are poor prenatal care foetal abuse, precipitous labour or unassisted delivery, neonaticide, and/or post-partum emotional disturbance (Apfel and Handel, 1996).

In-patient care with integrated psychiatric and obstetric services has shown to improve perinatal outcome in women with chronic mental illness; sometimes, in-patient care may be needed. Indications for hospitalization include threats of violence towards the foetus, neglect of prenatal care due to delusions, inability to meet the special nutritional needs of pregnancy, risk of precipitous delivery, and attempts to prematurely self-deliver.

Discussions regarding her changing roles and additional responsibilities need to start early in the course of pregnancy. This will prepare the patient and give her time to adjust to her new roles. This will also help caregivers to detect any negative reactions towards the pregnancy or the anticipated problems. Wherever indicated and possible, temporary guardianship for the baby may need to be planned for.

### *Abortion*

Abortions are commoner in women with chronic mental illness than in women in the general population. Spontaneous abortions are commoner because of poor prenatal self-care, and medical terminations of pregnancy are commoner because of poor contraceptive practice and the high-risk for an unwanted pregnancy associated with an impaired capacity to care for the child.

Post-abortion psychological reactions are likely to be more severe in women with mental illness. This is true even if the abortion occurs with the consent of the patient. Following an abortion, the patient needs to mourn, and needs help to do so. She also needs help in a acknowledging her loss, and in planning for future contraception to prevent an unwanted pregnancy.

*Intranatal and Postnatal Concerns*

Severely psychotic women may ignore or may not express the experience of labour pains. As a result, early admission may be necessary to monitor the onset and progress of labour. Sometimes, even a well-prepared patient can harbour aggressive feelings towards her baby, or become anxious during actual childbirth, as there is a high incidence of recurrence or exacerbation of mental illness during the post-partum period (McNeil, 1987). Psychiatric deterioration has an impact on the mother-infant relationship. Acute symptoms after childbirth may include denial of childbirth, delusions that the baby is dead or abnormal, and hallucinations commanding the mother to harm the baby (Steward, 1984); these may provoke infanticide. Guilt may occur in women who realise that they are unable to care for their babies. Hence, supportive treatment should be constantly provided until well after delivery.

It can be difficult to treat the patient post-partum as the patient may refuse or postpone the needed hospitalization due to a lack of insight (often aggravated by the withholding of psychotropic medication during pregnancy) and a lack of mother-baby units in psychiatric facilities. The ability of a patient to take her baby home should be based on her mental state and on the presence of at least one other adult in the environment who can take care of both the mother and the child. The patient's mental state can be best assessed by observing mother-child interactions in the maternal units.

Guidance can be obtained from nursery staff and obstetric staff reports. Decisions should be guided by evidence of abilities for childcare in previous pregnancies. Hospitalization in psychiatric hospitals may facilitate bonding, or mourning for custody loss, or may permit more supervision and intervention when there is ambiguity (Steward and Gangbar, 1989).

The recent Andrea Yates case in the USA, where a severely mentally ill woman was convicted of harming her three children points to the inadequacy of care for post-partum mothers with SMI even in developed countries. Aggression and negative reactions to the chilld may be part of the psychiatric illness that need to be monitored and assessed regularly and interventions provided for the well being of the infant and mother ( Chandra *et al.*, 2002).

## Practical Issues Related to Parenting

Proper parenting is vital for the normal intellectual, emotional, and physical development of the child. The parenting abilities of women with chronic mental illness can be enhanced by the availability of support from the primary family, medical facilities (including psychiatrists, gynaecologists, and paediatricians), and tertiary organisations. Appropriate guidance should be available to the patient to help her care for her child and attend to its medical needs. The mother-child units should be monitored for early signs of neglect or abuse (Apfel and Handel, 1996).

Illness characteristics impair parenting skills. For instance, schizophrenic patients have a reduced ability to discern non-verbal cues as well as a compromised capacity to recognise affects from facial expressions; these deficits can impair mother-child interactions (Corrigan and Green, 1993). As compared with healthy mothers who are not mentally ill, schizophrenic mothers touch less and play less with children (Gamer *et al.*, 1976), and exhibit withdrawal or inappropriate involvement (Abernethy and Grunebaum, 1972). Treatment with antipsychotics drugs can complicate matters because these drugs may decrease spontaneity (Nicholson and Blanch, 1994).

Some problems in parenting may arise from offspring characteristics. Children of schizophrenic mothers may be 'difficult' and slow to warm up. Contact with the separation from their mothers both have the potential to disturb normal emotional development in these children. If parenting is adequate, it is probably advisable to leave the child with its mother (Walker and Emory, 1983).

Problems in parenting may also arise from practical aspects of living. Homelessness among mentally ill mothers is common. This problem requires the attention of governmental and non-governmental organisations so that group homes or houses for such mothers may be made available (Nicholson *et al.*, 1993; Goering *et al.*, 1992). Unemployment and financial difficulties are also common among mentally ill mothers; they may require assistance with money management (O' Hara, 1986). These matters thus become necessary elements in rehabilitation programmes.

Programmes may be necessary to enhance a patient's parenting skills. These programmes need to be individually tailored with the patient's assets and liabilities in mind. Emphasis should be laid on self-reliance and on enhancement of self-esteem; both can improve confidence in parenting. Several model programmes have been developed (Waldo *et al.*, 1987) that teach parenting skills to schizophrenic mothers, monitors the developmental progress of the children, and allows for early intervention if needed. The programme provides developmental education to promote awareness of possible developmental delays, and to allay anxieties about the child's development. The programme also teaches good communication skills techniques for contraception. Themes which can be addressed in the programme are—the effects of illness on parenting, and maternal feelings of ambivalence.

## Major Mental Illness and Sexuality

Women with major mental illness have the same kind of sexual fantasies, urges and feelings, and face the same problems related to sexuality that healthy women do (Apfel and Handel, 1996). There is, therefore, a felt need for caregivers to address these matters. Several additional issues also assume importance in patients with major mental illness. Certain of these concerns are dealt with in the sections that follow.

### *General Sexual Knowledge and Behaviour*

Women with schizophrenia may have many misunderstandings about sexual anatomy and physiology, and may lack the basic vocabulary for discussing sex; discussions about sexuality may consequently prove difficult in such patients (Rozensky and Berman, 1984; Kalichman *et al.*, 1994). In a study of schizophrenic women, 52 per cent of subjects were found to have been sexually active during the previous 6 months; sexual activity was greater in women with greater psychopathology, in younger women, in women with lower levels of functioning, and in women with delusions (Kalichman *et al.*, 1994)

## High-Risk Behaviour

The prevalence of Human Immunodeficiency Virus (HIV) infection in persons with severe and persisting mental illness is 10-76 times greater than the rate found in the general population.

Data from the West indicate that 4-23 per cent of chronic mentally ill women are infected with HIV as compared with 0.3-0.4 per cent of women in the general population (Carey *et al.*, 1995; Weinhardt *et al.*, 1998a). Research has begun to examine HIV-related high-risk behaviour in mentally ill women. Studies among community-based samples have found a significant prevalence of high-risk sexual behaviours in women with long-standing schizophrenia; such behaviours include having multiple sexual partners, engaging in sex for money, and participating in homosexual encounters. For example, in a study of 47 chronic mentally ill women in New York, Cournos *et al.* (1994) found that 29 per cent reported having had multiple sexual partners, 21 per cent reported having been involved in coercive sex, and 9 per cent reported having had sex with intravenous drug-users during the previous year. These women were, in general, unlikely to use condoms. A history of sexually transmitted diseases was present in many women, as also history of current alcohol and drug use in conjunction with sex. Many women reported sexual contacts with unfamiliar persons, such as persons encountered in bars and psychiatric clinics. Many women were also often involved in sex in exchange of money or drugs. There were no differences in risk behaviour between women diagnosed with paranoid schizophrenia, other schizophrenic categories, schizoaffective disorder, or bipolar disorder.

Studying 61 women with severe mental illness in the USA, Weinhardt *et al.* (1998a) found that 54 per cent had been sexually active during the past 2 months; 38 per cent reported at least one of the following risk factors during that period: having more than one male partner; having anonymous male partner(s); having intercourse without a condom with a known or suspected polygamous partner; having sex with a person after alcohol or drug use; having sex with a parenteral drug user; trading sex for money, drugs or lodging; being forced into sex; and/or, receiving drugs of addiction by a parenteral route. Twenty-three per cent of the sample reported two or more of these risk factors, and 16 per cent reported three or more risk factors. Among those with multiple sexual partners, condom use was rare.

In a study from India, Chopra *et al.*, (1998) reported high-risk sexual behaviour among nearly 20 per cent of women psychiatric patients in Bangalore, India. Many patients had experienced sexual abuse; many patients also expressed an inability to insist on safe sex in their partners and spouses. A recent study conducted in NIMHANS, Bangalore among psychiatric inpatients has found the prevalence of high risk sexual behavior among women to be as high as 6 per cent (Chandra *et al.*, in press). The study was carried out to investigate the prevalence and correlates of sexual risk behaviour among psychiatric inpatients in India. Consecutive inpatients ($n = 618$) were assessed using a structured interview and standardized measures. Women were more likely to be sexually active (50%) than men (36%), but less likely (11% *vs* 20%) to engage in risky behaviour. Common risk behaviours included having a risky partner, having multiple partners, and exchanging money for sex. Being sexually active was associated with younger age, being married, being diagnosed with a disorder other than schizophrenia, and a history of drug use problems. However, the prevalence of these risk behaviours varied by gender. Women were more likely to report a history of a sexually transmitted infection (58%) or having exchanged sex for money (27%) whereas men were likely to report exchanging money for sex (66%). Of the 125 patients who reported risky sexual behaviour, 23 (18%) reported only one risk factor, 48 (38%) reported two, and 54 (43%) reported more than two risk factors.

These studies clearly indicate that identifying and combating high-risk behaviour in sexually active mentally ill women is an important issue all over the world.

### *Knowledge about and Attitudes Towards HIV Infection*

It is necessary to study female patients' knowledge about and attitudes towards HIV infection as this information would help in the development of appropriate management strategies. In a study on this subject, Weinhardt *et al.*, (1998a) found that women with chronic mental illness rated insufficient money, unemployment, relationship problems, transportation needs, psychiatric care, and health care as more serious concerns than the risk for HIV infection.

Though patients with severe mental illness may have a reasonable basic knowledge about HIV transmission and the methods of prevention thereof, several misconceptions may exist: a common misconception is that confidentiality about an HIV positive test will not be maintained. Misconceptions can interfere with important HIV-preventive behaviours. Even in the absence of misconceptions, individuals with adequate information and the necessary motivation to engage in HIV preventive behaviour may not do so due to deficits in safe sex negotiation skills, or the fear of loss of an emotionally or financially supportive relationship.

## **Management of High-Risk Behaviour**

### *General Issues*

The following general issues need to be kept in mind when managing women with long-standing mental illness:

1. Like healthy women, these women have sexual needs, and require to learn how to express their sexuality in a safe way.

2. High-risk behaviour in mentally ill women usually occurs in the context of limited knowledge, unawareness of personal risks, or the existence of other concerns which override the concern for guarding against HIV infection.
3. Mentally ill women may experience symptoms such as hyper-sexuality, impulsivity, and poor judgement; these can compromise the likelihood of safe sex.
4. Mentally ill women often lack the assertive skills necessary to have safe sex.
5. Unstable and transient interpersonal relationships can predispose to high-risk behaviour in mentally ill women.
6. Mentally ill women are often forced into sex; this compromises their ability to guard against HIV infection.
7. Mentally ill women and their partners may use alcohol or drugs before sex; this lessens the likelihood that safe sex will be practiced.

## Education

In general, when educating patients about sex, it is necessary to discuss aspects of sexuality as well as the risk of HIV infection; care must be taken to teach methods for the practice of safe sex. Sex education of this nature has been imparted to schizophrenic patients with successful short-term results (Berman and Rozensky, 1984; Kalichman *et al.*, 1995). However, unless the desired behaviour is reinforced or contextualized, the acquired knowledge and skills decay over time (Kalichman *et al.*, 1995).

Often, it is necessary to provide appropriate education to health-care staff as well. In an in-patient unit or in a community setting, the staff may ignore some obvious or inappropriate intimacies that arise between the patients (Cournos *et al.*, 1990). Cohen and Tanenbaum (1985) developed an interdisciplinary sex education programme for staff in long-term psychiatric hospitals. The programme sought to enhance comfortable discussions about sexuality and patient care, to guide personnel in the assessment of risk behaviour, and facilitate their ability to implement intervention strategies.

When educating patients, information regarding HIV transmission, risk behaviours and risk situations, condom use and the effectiveness thereof, the course of HIV infection, consequences of HIV infection, and issues related to HIV testing need to be communicated. Misconceptions, which may prevent risk-reducing behaviours, need to be identified and addressed. Risk sensitization can be encouraged through the presentation of a videotaped interview of a local woman infected with HIV. Motivation for the practice of safe sex should be encouraged. Personalized education must be provided rather than a standard package of information with do's and don'ts.

### Acquisition of Self-Management Skills

Patients should learn self-management skills, such as how to buy, keep, and use condoms. They should learn to identify the high-risk situations in which they are vulnerable to unprotected sex; for example, patients are less likely to take precautions if they have sex alter using alcohol or illicit drugs, if they have sex during periods of anxiety or depression, or if they venture into situations in which they are likely to be coerced into sex. Fears about or negative attitudes towards the implementation of various safe sex measures should be identified and tackled; for example, some women may be anxious about their partners' response should they insist on the use of a condom. Motivational issues should be addressed.

### Acquisition of Assertive Skills

Women with severe mental illness typically have extensive social skills deficits (Dilk and Bond, 1996); sexual assertive skills training may therefore help these women reduce their risk for HIV infection. Such assertive training can help women learn how to persuade unwilling male partners to use a condom.

Assertive training can be accomplished through simulated interactions by the group facilitators, participant practice and instructive feedback. The generalization of acquired skills to actual sexual interactions needs to be monitored. The importance of sexual assertiveness is recognised by leading theoretical models of risk-taking such as the information-motivation-behavioural skills model (Fisher and Fisher, 1992). According to this model, a deficit in sexual assertiveness skills hinders risk-reduction efforts in a woman who is motivated to change her behaviour; this is because the woman finds it difficult to negotiate for safer sex behaviour with her partner.

A study incorporating these management methods showed that women with chronic mental illness can acquire and maintain the information and skills needed to reduce their chances of infection with HIV. Treated women enhanced their sexual assertiveness skills and maintained this improvement over a 4-month follow-up period (Weinhardt *et al.*, 1998b).

**Other Significant Issues**

Management programmes should attempt to modify the social context in which high-risk behaviour occurs. Special contexts are those related to vulnerable interpersonal relationships, substance abuse, and sexual abuse. Women may be reluctant to initiate a conversation about condoms because of the fear that this may result in an aggressive confrontation, injury, or the end of the relationship; realistic risk-reducing practices therefore need to be built within these contexts. Chronic mental illnesses are often comorbid with drug and alcohol abuse disorders (Regier *et al.*, 1990). Alcohol and drug use prior to risky sex may be common among adults with a chronic mental illness (Carey *et al.*, 1997). Therefore, the association between the use of alcohol and illicit drugs on the one hand and unsafe sexual behaviour on the other hand needs to be addressed. Whether this association is direct or results from a third variable such as impulsivity requires exploration. Sexual abuse is more common among women with chronic mental illness than in the general population (Rosenberg *et al.*, 1996);

interventions need to be developed to address this problem. Patients should be helped to break abusive relationships. Referral to domestic abuse shelters should be made if such facilities are available.

Finally, therapists should encourage patients to seek testing if there is a, history of unprotected anal or viginal intercourse with a partner whose HIV serostatus is unknown or positive, or if there is a history of substance abuse using shared needles. Depending on the client's level of functioning, therapists should consider assisting with the scheduling of the test and coordinating counselling efforts with the testing site. With the prospect of testing, clients may experience an increase in anxiety and other psychiatric symptoms. Intensive therapist support, increased attention to suicidal ideation and, possibly, increased pharmacotherapeutic cover may be necessary for some clients.

## Major Mental Illness and Gynaecological Care

### *General Issues*

Women with major mental illness require gynaecological care as do all other women; mental health professionals should regularly assess the need for such care because many patients may never seek assistance even if the need arises. A good reproductive history should be obtained at the initial contact with the patient, and symptoms related to the reproductive system should be asked after during the first, and at all subsequent consultations. Appropriate gynaecological care should be negotiated for depending on the need (D'Ercole *et al.,* 1991). Implementation of the gynaecologist's recommendations should be monitored (Handel, 1985). Preventive measures should be undertaken as required, such as counselling about regular breast examination for suspicious lumps, annual cervical smear examinations after the age of 40, and annual mammograms after the age of 50.

The institution of such measures of care conveys to both patients and staff that a woman's concerns about her body are important. For women with chronic mental illness, for whom much of the treatment is genderless and focused on thought and behaviour, visits to the gynaecologist can become a place to discuss concerns about their bodies.

*Family Planning*

The family planning needs of women with chronic mental illness should be understood in relation to the outcome of pregnancy in these women. Coverdale and Aruffo (1989) found that 33 per cent of patients who were sexually active did not want to become pregnant, yet did not use birth control methods; 31 per cent of patients had at least one abortion to terminate an unwanted pregnancy, and 60 per cent of the babies born to these patients were being reared by people other than the mothers. These data indicate that women with chronic mental illness may require counselling services for family planning and contraception because they experience difficulties in coping with the stress of parenthood. Most health professionals agree that suitable family planning information should be provided to women with mental illness (Coverdale *et al.*, 1992).

Grunebaum *et al.* (1971) found that most female patients preferred to obtain family planning counselling in mental health settings. Follow-up studies of patients who received such counselling in psychiatric hospitals have shown that most patients continue contraception after discharge, and many patients upgrade to safer, more effective methods of contraception (Abernethy *et al.*, 1975). Yet, despite the need and the desire for services with demonstrated efficacy, the provision of family planning counselling in mental health settings is relatively rare. As a striking example, Rudolph *et al.* (1990) observed that family planning and contraceptive measures were not mentioned in most charts of women with psychotic disorders who were hospitalized during pregnancies.

Offering family planning services together with mental health services has many advantages. The first advantage is one of convenience: women with chronic mental illness may find it hard to tackle the practical problems associated with attending separate psychiatric and family planning clinics; in fact, for many women, the psychiatrist may be the only contact with the health care system. The second advantage relates to consent: during periods of mental stability, women can provide their psychiatrists with an advance informed consent for interventions related to various reproductive events that may occur during a psychotic period. The third advantage is related to skills training: mental health professionals are in an ideal position to offer skills training on how to reduce unwanted sex and how to practice safe sex.

Family planning counselling should therefore provide information about the heritability of the illness; about the side effects and teratogenecity of drugs so that patients can then make better informed decisions about family planning (Packer, 1992). It must be kept in mind that women with bipolar illness may minimize the burden of their illness and deny the possibility that it could be inherited (Targum *et al.*, 1981).

*Guidelines for Family Planning Services*

Coverdale *et al.*, (1992) have provided practical guidelines for family planning services for women with chronic mental illness. First, a meticulous history should be obtained about sexual behaviour and experiences, pregnancies, and ability to care for children. Next, education about various contraceptive methods should be provided; it must, however, be kept in mind that patients with cognitive deficits or thought disorder will have impaired ability to use such information. Therefore, an attempt should also be made to discuss family planning with the patients' sexual partners. Wherever necessary and feasible, sexual assertiveness training should also be provided to the patients.

Some practical problems may arise these must be identified and tackled. For example, women with chronic mental illness often do not take their pills as scheduled; oral contraceptives may therefore be an unsuitable method for contraception. Oral contraceptives may also induce mood changes, potentially leading to impaired drug compliance. Schizophrenics have an increased threshold for pain and may not recognise or admit early symptoms of pelvic inflammation; the use of intrauterine devices may therefore be associated with medical risks (Bacharch, 1985). Sometimes, contraceptive implants and intrauterine devices may become a focus of delusions of control (Coverdale *et al.*, 1993). Barrier methods of contraception may be unwise considering the high likelihood of unplanned and pressured sex among women with schizophrenia (Miller and Finnerty, 1996), and the difficulties that schizophrenic women experience in negotiating with their partners for the use of such methods; however, condom us has the advantage of conferring protection against HIV infection.

## Violence in Women with Severe Mental Illness

The Disabled Women's Network of Canada (Ridington, 1989) surveyed 245 women with disabilities and found that 40 per cent had experienced abuse; 12 per cent had been raped. Perpetrators of the abuse were primarily spouses and ex-spouses (37%) and strangers (28%), followed by parents (15%), service providers (10%), and dates (7%). Less than half these experiences were reported, due mostly to fear and dependency. Ten per cent of the women had used shelters or other services, 15 per cent reported that no services were available or they were unsuccessful in their attempts to obtain services, and 55 per cent had not tried to get services.

Sobsey and Doe (1991) conducted a study of 166 abuse cases handled by the University of Alberta's Sexual Abuse and Disability Project. The sample was 82 per cent women and 70 per cent persons with intellectual impairments, and covered a very wide age range (18 months to 57 years). In 96 per cent of the cases, the perpetrator was known to the victim; 44 per cent of the perpetrators were service providers. Seventy-nine per cent of the individuals were victimized more than once. Treatment services were either inadequate or not offered in 73 per cent of the cases.

An exploratory study from Bangalore sought (*a*) to determine the prevalence of sexual coercion in a representative sample of female psychiatric patients in India, (*b*) to identify clinical and sociodemographic correlates of sexual coercion, (*c*) to clarify the association between sexual coercion and HIV-related risk behaviour, and (*d*) to determine whether self-report of sexual coercion from these patients was recorded in their medical charts ( Chandra *et al.,* in press).

To address these issues, consecutive female inpatient admissions ($n = 146$) to a large psychiatric hospital in southern India were assessed using a structured interview and standardized measures. During structured clinical interviews, sexual coercion was reported by as high as 30 per cent of the 146 women. The most commonly reported experience involved sexual intercourse involving threatened or actual physical force (reported by 14% of women), and the most commonly identified perpetrator was the woman's husband or intimate partner (15%), or a person in a position of authority in their community (10%). Women with a history of abuse were more likely to report HIV-related sexual behaviour. In contrast to the 30 per cent of women who reported sexual coercion during interviews, only 3.5 per cent of the medical records contained this information. These results indicate that sexual coercion is a serious and prevalent concern among female Indian psychiatric patients, but is rarely reported in medical charts. Increased screening and reporting are indicated, as are sexual abuse prevention and treatment programs.

There have been virtually no studies that examine the existence, feasibility, or effectiveness of abuse interventions for women with disabilities. In both the disability rights movement and the battered women's movement, it is generally acknowledged that programmes to assist abused women are often architecturally inaccessible and are not able to accommodate women who need assistance with daily self-care or medications. Crisis interventions typically include escaping temporarily to a woman's shelter, having an escape plan ready in the event of imminent violence if the woman chooses to remain with the perpetrator, and escaping permanently from the abuser. These options may be problematic for the woman with a disability if the shelter is inaccessible or unable to meet her needs for personal assistance with activities of daily living, if the shelter staff are unable to communicate with a deaf or speech-impaired woman, if she depends primarily on the abuser for assistance with personal needs and has no family or friends to stay with, or if she is physically incapable of executing the tasks necessary to implement an escape plan such as packing necessities, hiding money, and driving or arranging transportation to a shelter or friend's home.

There are several requirements for effective victim services for women with mental illnesses and intellectual impairments. First, service providers need to provide adequate assessment of survivors, including questions about disability-related issues. Second, abuse service providers should be trained to recognise and effectively respond to needs related to the disability, and disability service providers should be trained in recognising and responding to physical and sexual trauma. Third, barriers to services should be eliminated by providing barrier-free information and referral services, by ensuring physical accessibility to facilities, by providing 24-hour access to transportation, to interpreters, and to communication assistance, and by providing trained personnel to monitor risks and respond to victims receiving services through disability programmes. Finally, women with mental illness, who are dependent on caregivers, either at home or in institutions, may need special legal protection against abuse.

## In Conclusion

All issues related to women are also applicable to women with mental illness. Illness, however, amplifies many issues and creates new ones. Therefore, special attention needs to be paid to the special, gender-based needs of women with major mental illness. Good mental health care should therefore integrate aspects related to sexuality, reproduction, and parenting into the management package in order to lessen the adverse consequences for women as well as children. Various phases in a woman's life, such as the pre-menstrual period, pregnancy, the post-partum period, and menopause, need special consideration with regard to both psychosocial and pharmacological management. Women recovering from mental illness need support for legal issues. They need to be protected from violence to which they are highly prone and services tailored to their needs must exist in all shelters and cells dealing with violence. It is important that professionals working with women in various sectors are trained to identify and cater to the needs of women who are living with a severe mental illness, to ensure that they do not remain invisible forever.

## REFERENCES

Abernethy, V.D. and Grunebaum, H. (1972): 'Towards a Family Planning Programme in Psychiatric Hospitals', *Am J. Public Health:* 62: 1638-45.

Abernethy V.D., Grunebaum H., Groover B. *et al.*, (1975): 'Contraceptive Continuation of Hospitalized Psychiatric Patients', *Family Planning Perspectives.*

Apfel, R. and Handel, M. (1996): 'Women with Long-Term Mental Illness: A Different Voice', in Soreff S.M. (ed.), *Handbook for the Treatment of the Severely Mentally Ill.* Seattle: Hogarge and Huber: 326-49.

Bachrach, L.L. (1985): 'Chronic Mentally Ill Women: Emergence and Legitimization of Programme Issues', *Hospital Community Psychiatry:* 36: 1063-9.

Bernam, C. and Rozensky, R.H. (1984): 'Sex Education for the Chronic Psychiatric Patient: The Effect of Sexual Issues Group on Knowledge and Attitudes', *Psychosoc. Rehab.* J.: 8: 28-34.

Carey, M.P., Weinhardt L.S. and Carey, K.B. (1995): 'Prevalence of Infection with HIV Among the Serious Mentally Ill: Review of Research and Implications for Practice', *Prof. Psychol. Res. Prac:* 26: 262-8.

Carey, M.P., Carey, K.B. and Kalichman, S.C. (1997): 'Risk for Human Immunodeficiency Virus (HIV) Infection Among Persons with Severe Mental Illness', *Clin, Psychol. Review:* 17: 271-91.

Chandra, P.S. and Vijaylakshmi, K. (2000): 'Major Mental Illness in Women: Clinical Issues' in C. Andrade (ed), *Advances in Psychiatry.* New Delhi: Oxford University Press: 185-214.

Chandra, P.S., Venkatsubramaniam, G., and Thomas, T. (2002): 'Infanticidal Ideas and Infanticidal Behaviour In Severe Postpartum Psychiatric Disorders', *Journal of Nervous and Mental Disease:* 190: 457-461.

Chandra P.S., Carey, M.P., Carey, K.B., Shalinianant and Thomas T—(In Press): 'Sexual Coercion and Abuse Among Women with a Severe Mental Illness in India: An Exploratory Investigation', *Comprehensive Psychiatry.*

Chandra, P.S., Carey, M.P., Carey, K.B., .Prasada Rao, PSDV, Jairam K. R., and Tinku Thomas (In Press): 'HIV Risk Behaviour among Psychiatric Inpatients: Results from a Hospital-Wide Screening Study in Southern India', *International Journal of STD and AIDS.*

Chopra, M.P., Savitha Sri E.V. and Chandra, P.S. (1998): 'HIV-Related Risk Among Psychiatric Inpatients From India', *Psychiatr. Serv:* 49: 823-5

Cohen, D. and Tanenbaum, R. (1985): 'Sexuality Education for Staff in Long-Term Psychiatric Hospitals', *Hospital Community Psychiatry:* 36: 187-9.

Corrigan, P. W. and Green, M.F. (1993): 'Schizophrenic Patients, Sensitivity to Social Cues: The Role of Abstraction', *Am. J. Psychiatry:* 150: 589-94.

Cournos, F., Guido, J.R., Coomaraswamy S., Meyer-Bahlburg H., Sugden, R. and Horwath, E. (1994): 'Sexual Activity and Risk of HIV Infection Among Patients with Schizophrenia', *Am. J. Psychiatry:* 151: 228-32.

Coverdale, J.H. and Aruffo, J.A. (1989): 'Family Planning Needs of Female Chronic Psychiatric Outpatients', *Am. J. Psychiatry:* 146: 1489-91.

Coverdale, J.H., Aruffo, J.A. and Grunebaum, H. (1992): 'Developing Family Planning Services for Female Chronic Mentally Ill Outpatients', *Hospital Community Psychiatry:* 43: 475-8.

Coverdale, J.H., Bayer, T.L., McCullough, L.B. *et al.*, (1993): 'Respecting the Autonomy of Chronic Mentally Ill Women in Decisions about Contraception', *Hospital Community Psychiatry:* 44: 671-6.

Dilk, M.N. and Bond, G.R. (1996): 'Meta-Analytic Evaluation of Skills Training Research for Individuals with Severe Mental Illness', *J. Consult. Clin. Psychol.:* 64: 1337-46.

D'Ercole, A., Skodol, A.E., Stuening, E. *et al.*, (1991): 'Diagnosis of Physical Illness in Psychiatric Patients Using Axis III and a Standardized Medical History', *Hospital Community Psychiatry:* 42: 395-400.

Fisher, J.D. and Fisher, W.A. (1992): 'Changing AIDS-Related Risk Behaviour', *Psychol. Bull.:* 111: 455-74.

Gamer, E., Gallant D. and Grunebaum, H. (1976): 'Children of Psychitic Mothers: an Evaluation of 1-Year Olds on Test of Object Permanence', *Arch. Gen. Psychiatry:* 33:311-17.

Goering, P., Wasylenki, D., St. Onge, M. *et al.*, (1992): 'Gender Differences Among Clients of a Case Management Program for the Homeless,' *Hospital Community Psychiatry:* 43: 160-5.

Grunebaum, H.U., Abernethy, V.D., Rofman, E.S. *et al.,* (1971): 'The Family Planning Attitudes, Practices and Motivations of Mental Patients', *Am. J Psychiatry:* 128: 740-4.

Handel M. (1985): 'Deferred Pelvic Examinations: A Purposeful Omission in the Care of Mentally Ill Women', *Hospital Community Psychiatry:* 36: 1070-4.

Kalichman, S.C., Kelly J.A, Johnson J.R. *et al.,* (1994): 'Factors Associated with Risk for HIV Infection Among Chronic Mentally Ill Adults', *Am. J. Psychiatry:* 151: 221-7.

Kalichman, S.C., Sikkema K.J., Kelly J.A. *et al.,* (1995): 'Use of a Brief Behavioural Skills Intervention to Prevent HIV Infection Among Chronic Mentally Ill Adults', *Psychiatry:* 150: 60-8.

McNeil, T.F. (1987): 'A Prospective Study of Postpartum Psychoses in a High-Risk Group: 2. Relationships to Demographic and Psychiatric History Characteristics', *Acta. Psychiatr. Scand.:* 75: 35-43.

Miller, L.J. (1990): 'Psychotic Denial of Pregnancy: Phenomenology and Clinical Management', *Hospital Community Psychiatry:* 41: 1233-7.

Miller, L.J. and Finnerty, M. (1996): 'Sexuality, Pregnancy and Child Rearing Among Women with Shizophrenia Spectrum Disorders', *Psychiatr. Serv.:* 47: 502-5.

Miller Jr. W.H., Bloom, J.D. and Resnick, M.P. (1992): 'Prenatal Care for Pregnant Chronic Mentally Ill Patients', *Hospital Community Psychiatry:* 43: 942-3.

Nicholson, J. and Balnch, A. (1994): 'Rehabilitation for Parenting Roles for People with Serious Mental Illness', *Psychosoc. Rehab J.:* 18: 109-19.

Nicholson, J., Geller, J., Fisher, W.H. *et al.,* (1993): 'State Policies and Programs that Address the Needs of Mentally Ill Mothers in the Public Sector', *Hospital Community Psychiatry:* 44: 484-9.

O'Hara, M.W. (1986): 'Social Support, Life Events and Depression During Pregnancy and the Puerperium', *Arch. Gen. Psychiatry:* 43: 569-73.

Packer, S. (1992): 'Family Planning for Women with Bipolar Disorder', *Hospital Community Psychiatry:* 43: 479-82.

Regier, D., Farmer, M., Rae, D. *et al.,* (1990): 'Co-Morbidity of Mental Disorders with Alcohol and Other Drug Abuse: Results from the Epidemiologic Catchment Area Study', *JAMA:* 264: 2511-18.

Ridington, J. (1989): 'Beating The 'Odds': Violence and Women With Disabilities' (Position Paper 2),Vancouver, Canada, Disabled Women's Network.

Rosenberg, S.D., Darke, R.E. and Mueser, K. (1996): 'New Directions for Treatment Research of Sexual Abuse in Persons with Severe Mental Illness', *Community Mental Health Journal:* 32: 387-400.

Rozensky, R.H. and Berman, C. (1984): 'Sexual Knowledge, Attitudes and Experiences of Chronic psychiatric patients', *Psychosocial Rehab Journal:* 8: 21-7.

Sobsey, D., Wells, D., Lucardie, R., and Mansell, S. (eds) (1995): *Violence and Disability: An Annotated Bibliography,* Baltimore, MD: Paul H. Brookes.

Steward, D. E. (1984): 'Pregnancy And Schizophrenia', *Can. Fam. Physician:* 30: 1537-41.

Steward, D.E. and Gangbar, R. (1989): 'Psychiatric Assessment of Competency to Care for a Newborn', *Can. J. Psychiatry:* 34: 34-8.

Targum S.D., Dibble, E.D., Davenport, Y.B. *et al.,* (1981): 'The Family Attitude Questionnaire: Patients and Spouses Views of Bipolar Illness', *Arch. Gen. Psychiatry:* 38: 562-8.

Waldo, M.C., Roath, M., Levine, W. *et al.,* (1987): 'A Model Program to Teach Parenting Skills to Schizophrenic Mothers', *Hospital Community Psychiatry:* 38: 1110-12.

Weinhardt, L.S., Carey, M.P. and Carey, K.B. (1998a): 'HIV Risk Behaviour and the Public Health Context of HIV/AIDS Among Women Living with a Severe and Persistent Mental Illness', *J. Nerv. Ment. Dis.:* 186: 276-82.

Weinhardt, L.S., Carey, M.P. and Carey, K.B. *et al.,* (1998b): 'Increasing Assertiveness Skills To Reduce HIV Risk Among Women with a Severe and Persistent Mental Illness', *J. Consult. Clin. Psychol.:* 66: 680-4.

5

# MENTAL HEALTH MATTERS TOO

## Gynaecological Symptoms and Depression in Goa

*Vikram Patel*

Reproductive health, in its broadest definition, has been described as a fundamental and inalienable part of women's health and includes issues as varied as sexuality and women's empowerment. While it has been suggested that mental health is also a component of reproductive health (Ford Foundation, 1997), this remains, at best, a peripheral and marginal concern. The areas of intersection of reproductive and mental health are considerable in scope. If one were to enumerate specific areas of overlap, the list would include the psychological issues related to childbirth, violence, rape, adverse maternal outcomes such as stillbirths and miscarriage, surgery on and removal of reproductive organs, sterilization, pre-marital pregnancies in adolescents, HIV/AIDS and the impact of menopause and infertility. These issues are vast in range and cannot be addressed in one article.

This paper will examine the relationship of depression, the most common mental health problem in women, with the complaint of vaginal discharge, the most common reproductive health complaint in women, with a focus on the literature from South Asia. The article is based on a review of the published literature on gynaecological morbidity and mental disorders from South Asia. This article serves to explore the potential association between these two, apparently unrelated, health problems and, using the existing literature, presents a hypothesis that one key factor accounting for the high rate of non-specific, self-reported complaints is depression. Finally, the article will present briefly the preliminary data arising from a cohort study in progress in Goa which is investigating this hypothesis.

**Women and Depression: The Burden of Mental Illness**

Depression and anxiety disorders are by far the most common psychological illnesses in the world. While current classification systems in psychiatric research tend to view these disorders as distinct categories, in reality they are closely related to one another and are often lumped together under the older term of neuroses or the term now in vogue: 'common mental disorders' (Goldberg *et al.*, 1992). For the sake of semantic simplicity, the term 'depression' is used in this article. The *World Health Report* based on 1993 statistics shows that depression is the third most frequent cause of morbidity (prevalence rates) worldwide (WHO, 1995). The Global Burden of Disease[4] (Murray *et al.*, 1996) reports that of the ten leading causes of disability worldwide, five were neuropsychiatric disorders. Of these, depression was the most common and accounted for more than one in ten years of life lived with disability. The evidence of a high prevalence of depression has been generated from a range of settings in low-income countries including primary health care settings in Goa (Patel *et al.*, 1998). These studies reveal prevalence figures of depression approaching 20-25 per cent in women in the community and up to 40 per cent of adult primary care populations.

The high prevalence of depression is of concern for many reasons. There is convincing evidence of a relationship between depression and disability independent of any co-existing physical illness (Ormal *et al.*, 1994). Additionally, there is the association of such disorders with economic deprivation, such as being unemployed, being in debt or belonging to the lower income groups of society (Patel *et al.*, 1999). Thus, those who are already vulnerable due to their disadvantaged economic circumstances risk becoming ill with a disorder which will further disable them and render them less able to cope with adverse circumstances that they already faced. Finally, despite the above evidence, most individuals with depression remain undiagnosed and untreated. In many developing countries, persons with depression are treated with a range of symptomatic medicines such as analgesics for aches and pains, 'tonics' and vitamin injections for fatigue and tiredness, and sleeping pills for insomnia (Patel *et al.*, 1998, Linden *et al.*, 1999). Patients are typically subjected to numerous costly investigations and polypharmacy and consult many health practitioners in an attempt to gain relief from their illness. Rarely are any structured counselling therapies or antidepressants used; in most countries the latter are not even on the essential drugs list and thus remain unavailable to patients in public health care settings.

From the perspective of reproductive health, the key epidemiological finding on depression is the much-replicated association with gender. Both community-based studies and studies of treatment seekers indicate that women are disproportionately affected by depression. The obvious questions thrown up by this finding are the reason for this apparent vulnerability, and its significance. Davar has reviewed this issue in detail in a recent book (Davar, 1999). There is considerable evidence demonstrating that stressful life events are closely associated with depression and such events are more common in the lives of women. Thus, women are far more likely to be victims of violence in their homes. Differences may also be partly accounted for by a gender bias in the way mental problems are diagnosed, since these are often influenced by cultural expectations and stereotypes of what is normal behaviour for men and women. Because of the different expectations and evaluations of men's and women's behaviour, mental illness in women may attract a greater amount of shame and dishonour and has a greater impact on family life due to the woman's role in running the domestic activities of the household. Women with mental health problems are less likely to receive appropriate health care when sick and when they do seek help, a gender bias ensures that symptoms are taken less seriously than they are for men. One area of health care, which, however, is gender-sensitive not least because of its specific emphasis on women's health, is gynaecological health care. Is there a link between women's gynaecological symptoms and depression?

**Reproductive Tract Symptoms and Infections: Evidence of Discordance**

Symptoms related to the reproductive tract are among the most common health problems in women in developing countries, particularly in South Asia. Community surveys have found that more than half of women report such complaints (Koenig *et al.*, 1998). The most common complaint is that of abnormal vaginal discharge; the recent NFHS-2 reported that about 1/3 of women reported this complaint at the time of the survey (IIPS, 2001). This complaint is typically associated as being due to reproductive tract infections (RTIs). Indeed, the WHO guidelines on the syndromic management of RTIs advocates the treatment of the complaint of abnormal vaginal discharge as if it were equivalent to a definitive RTI.

However, there is growing evidence that there is considerable discordance between a woman's self-reported gynaecological complaints and the existence of an RTI. A review of community surveys from South Asia reported that although 55 to 84 per cent of women have self-reported symptoms of gynaecological symptoms, about 26 to 74 per cent have clinically diagnosed conditions and that the rates of laboratory confirmed RTIs are even lower (Koenig *et al.*, 1998). The authors conclude that self-reported symptoms should not be considered as providing accurate estimates of the true prevalence of gynaecological morbidity in the community. A recent study with women attending a health centre with the complaint of vaginal discharge in Bangladesh, which employed the most sensitive laboratory tests for the diagnosis of RTIs found that 2 out of 3 women did not have an RTI (Hawkes *et al.*, 1999).

The overall conclusion is that the concordance between

self-reported symptoms and disease is, at best, weak; many women with the symptom have no disease and many women with the disease have no symptoms. Thus, at least half of complaints of vaginal discharge are 'medically unexplained'. A key question which emerges from this discordance is why women with no disease have the symptom. Clearly, one potential reason is the possibility of other gynaecological diseases or conditions such as the use of oral contraceptives. Methodological limitations in existing research, such as the use of vague questions about discharge and the failure to include questions about severity, may also lead to discordance. In addition, given the evidence quoted earlier of the high rates of depression in women, could some of this symptom burden be accounted for by psychological factors? Depression typically presents as medically unexplained physical symptoms such as tiredness, aches and pains, dizziness, palpitations and sleep problems. Such physical symptoms predict the onset of depression and *vice versa* and the co-existence of symptoms is associated with chronicity and the increased use of health services (Katon *et al.*, 1998, Hotopf *et al.*, 1998). Is there any evidence to support the hypothesis that depression and gynaecological morbidity, specifically vaginal discharge, are linked?

### Depression and Gynaecological Symptoms: The Evidence for a Link

There is a substantial literature from the West demonstrating a strong relationship between gynaecological symptoms and psychological disorders, in particular depression and anxiety (Gath *et al.*, 1987, Hodgkiss *et al.*, 1994). These studies show that the rates of psychological disorder in women with gynaecological symptoms are higher than the general population and that these rates are highest when there is no gynaecological pathology ('medically unexplained' symptoms). A review of the literature on psychiatric disorder in women attending gynaecological clinics found a mean prevalence of depressive disorder of nearly 50 per cent as compared to rates of 26 per cent in general medical clinic (Hunter, 1990). There is evidence that psychosocial factors play an important role in determining illness behaviour in women with gynaecological symptoms (*ibid*).

There is growing evidence now available from South Asia, much of it derived from qualitative research studies, which also demonstrates the co-morbidity of gynaecological and psychological illness, and specifically, the association of the complaint of vaginal discharge with mental stress and weakness. Higher rates of depression are reported in women attending gynaecological clinics. For example, a case-control study compared 120 women attending a gynaecology clinic for the first time with 55 women who reported no physical health problem. Half of the women in the former group were found to have a significant psychological disorder as compared to the expected figure of 26 per cent in the control group (Agarwal *et al.*, 1990). A study designed to explore the relationship between mental illness and gynaecological morbidity among low-income women in Mumbai found that half had at least one gynaecological symptom and about a quarter had a mental health problem. Both often co-existed, being most frequent in women aged 26-35 years (Blue *et al.*, 1995). In a qualitative study in rural Maharashtra, white discharge was mentioned as the most important and common problem in women. Local terminology for the discharge included the term *dhat,* which is similar to the local term for semen. Of the five types of discharge, which were recognised, the most common was a mild thin discharge, which was perceived to be caused by weakness. Probing of the term weakness elicited these symptoms: reduced sexual satisfaction, loss of energy, giddiness, tingling numbness in the extremities, lethargy, generalised aches and pains, loss of appetite, no desire to speak anything and gloomy mood (Bang *et al.*, 1996). These complaints are identical to the diagnostic symptoms of depression and anxiety. A qualitative study with 60 slum-dwelling women in Mumbai recorded an oppressive lifestyle for women:

'The majority of women stay at home where their

> movements and behaviour are closely supervised... women going out to work live in constant threat of violence... [the women] live cloistered defensive lives, their physical movements being severely restricted. The majority of husbands drink heavily and regularly beat their wives...there is very little communication between partners around daily lives and events'
>
> (IUSSP 1997).

Given that trauma, lack of social support and poor marital relationships are all life events whose association with depression is well established, this description paints a picture of a lifestyle which may be expected to lead to high rates of depression. Not surprisingly, then, weakness which was a common complaint, was often attributed by women to mental tension. Indeed, the authors found that mental stress is universally cited as among the most important problems women have, along with weakness. The main causes for mental stress cited by the women were poverty, husband's alcoholism, fears about the implications of vaginal discharge and unemployment of the husband.

## How are Depression and Gynaecological Morbidity Linked?

Somatisation is the process by which psychological disorders present with physical symptoms. Although once thought to be the characteristic form of presentation of depression in developing countries, it is now recognised that somatisation is the typical presentation in developed countries as well. A variety of theories are used to explain its mechanism (Hotopf *et al.*, 1998; Hunter 1990; Mumford 1993 and Patel *et al.*, 1998). Thus, somatic idioms are often used as metaphors for psychological distress (*e.g.* 'my heart is heavy'). Anxiety and depression can lead to changes in the autonomic nervous system leading to symptoms such as palpitations and muscle-tension related aches and pains. The stigma associated with complaining of psychosocial problems to biomedical professionals make the presentations of somatic symptoms less embarrassing. Depressed persons may be more likely to interpret normal physical sensations or experiences as being pathological. The literature on the specific association of somatisation in gynaecological and obstetric contexts is considerable and one journal (*Journal of Psychosomatic Obstetrics and Gynecology*) is devoted to this subject. Over the years, the journal has published an array of articles demonstrating the association between gynaecological complaints such as pelvic pain, menstrual irregularities and infertility with psychosocial factors and frank depressive disorders. Much of this literature was reviewed in a recent book on somatisation which included two chapters relevant to our discussion here. One chapter reviewed the psychosomatic basis of chronic pelvic pain (Pearce *et al.,* 1990), while the second examined the psychosomatic basis of gynaecological complaints (Hunter, 1990). The evidence showed that while symptoms were not always associated with pathology, the finding of pathology did not necessarily imply that it was the cause of the symptom. An interactive model of aetiology which incorporates physiological and psychosocial factors may provide a useful way of understanding this complex relationship. For example, pelvic pain may result from gynaecological diseases such as pelvic inflammatory disease, which in turn may lead to marital difficulties which are associated with depression. Depression, in turn, worsens the experience of the pain and delays recovery.

There is, by comparison, a very limited literature on somatisation in relation to gynaecological symptoms in India, most of it from Chaturvedi and colleagues in Bangalore (Chaturvedi *et al.,* 1993, Chaturvedi, 1998). In one study, the attributions of illness in 200 female psychiatric outpatients with physical symptoms were compared with 138 women who reported good health. A third of women in the former group attributed the cause of their symptoms to white vaginal discharge as compared to 13 per cent of the control group (Chaturvedi *et al.,* 1993). In another study, the psychiatric status of 70 women who presented with complaints of more than two somatic symptoms were studied. Women with identifiable major physical illnesses, menstrual irregularities, or gynaecological illness were excluded. Nearly half the women reported a white discharge and depression was more often diagnosed in these women (Chaturvedi, 1998). These studies support the notion that the complaint of white discharge in women may be analogous to the common complaint of semen discharge in men and, in the sense that it represents an explanatory model for psychosocial problems, it may represent a folk model of depression and anxiety. Thus, the complaint of vaginal discharge may represent the female equivalent of the well-defined psychosomatic condition in men in South Asia called the *Dhat* Syndrome (Malhotra *et al.*, 1975). This condition is characterised by complaints of seminal discharge associated with tiredness, anxiety and depression. The illness is linked to beliefs about the vitality of seminal fluid and thus, the potential association between its discharge and weakness. The reproductive somatic idiom in women may be adopted to seek help from medical professionals and to escape, albeit temporarily, from stressful situations. In extreme situations, women may adopt the sick role which legitimises a range of otherwise unacceptable behaviours such as the inability to perform household chores. There is also the possible linkage between gynaecological morbidity and its associated psychosocial determinants, such as violence and marital difficulties, leading to depression.

## Researching Gynaecological Morbidities and Mental Health

Although there is some evidence which points towards an association between gynaecological morbidity and psychosocial factors and depression, this can only be considered as tentative at this stage. There is clearly the need for systematic research which explores and describes the linkages between these two important public health issues. Such research needs to incorporate sensitive gold standard tests for the diagnosis of gynaecological causes of vaginal discharge, most importantly RTIs. After all, simply reporting an association between a physical symptom and depression has already been done and may have no greater import than the common finding that psychological illness often co-exists with physical illness. In order to examine whether depression is aetiologically linked to vaginal discharge, one would need to demonstrate that the rates of depression are higher in women with the complaint, but with no identifiable gynaecological disease (the 'medically unexplained' group). The demonstration that depression is a predictor of the development of gynaecological symptoms in a longitudinal study would further confirm this hypothesis. Evidence presented earlier also shows that many women with disease do not experience symptoms and that depression is associated with help-seeking behaviour in persons with physical health problems. Thus, another perspective for research is to examine the potential role of depression as a factor which influences help-seeking behaviour in women with RTIs.

A key area for any research investigation in mental health is examining its relationship with cultural factors. In many developing societies, depressive disorders are recognised as being distress states but are not understood in the same way as in EuroAmerican societies, *i.e.* the concepts about the causes and nature of the distress states may differ widely. Concepts such as depression, can be elicited in other societies, but may mean something quite different; for example, it may reflect the patients' assessment of their socio-economic and spiritual state. Thus, in many low-income societies depression is not viewed from a biomedical perspective (Patel *et al.*, 2001). Therefore, it is essential to generate a local language of depression and to explore its contextual significance and the explanatory models of the depressed individual; what the person believes is causing her distress, her understanding of the changes that are affecting her and how the distress has affected her daily life. There is an obvious role for the use of qualitative research methods in achieving these goals.

These are the precisely the objectives and scientific methods being employed in an ongoing community cohort study of gynaecological morbidity, reproductive tract infections and common mental disorders currently in progress in Goa. This study (Stree Arogya Shodh) began in October 2000 and is the result of a collaboration between the London School of

Hygiene and Tropical Medicine, the Sangath Society (a Goan NGO) and the Government of Goa's Directorate of Health Services. Three thousand women in the reproductive age group have been randomly selected to participate in a study in which each woman will be seen on three occasions over a 12 month period. On each occasion, data on her health will be collected and laboratory tests will be carried out. A sub-group of women with either vaginal discharge or depression or both are invited for serial in-depth interviews to explore the social and cultural contexts of these illness experiences. Prior to the main field study, piloting of the study methods was carried out including the first demonstration of the use of self-administered vaginal swabs in India (Tanksale *et al.*). At the time when this paper was presented, more than 1700 women had completed recruitment; from these women, data on 980 women had been cleaned and analysed. The early findings show that 21 per cent of women have an RTI; bacterial vaginosis and candidiasis are the commonest RTIs. 8 per cent of women suffer from a common mental disorder. Twenty per cent of women complain of abnormal vaginal discharge. In terms of the hypothesis we are testing, there was no association between women's complaints of discharge and their RTI status; however, women who complained of discharge were significantly more likely to be suffering from depression.

## Implications for Policy

If, indeed, the initial findings showing an association between vaginal discharge and depression are confirmed in the entire study, and particularly if we demonstrate a temporal relationship between depression and women's gynaecological complaints, the implications for policy and programmes are immense, given the scale of reported morbidity of both types of health problems. The inappropriate treatment and associated economic costs as a result of the symptom-based syndromic approach to gynaecological symptoms is now becoming apparent. The authors of the recent study from Bangladesh calculated that the application of the syndromic management approach led to high levels of over-treatment which, in turn, carried both financial and social costs, the latter in potentially exposing women misdiagnosed as having an RTI to threats of domestic disruption or even violence (Hawkes *et al.*, 1999). The description of the relationship between gynaecological symptoms and depression may provide the rationale for the development of more flexible models of reproductive health care which incorporate both physical symptoms and their psychosocial contexts. Evidence of the efficacy of such psychological interventions are already available from studies in South Asia (Patel *et al.*, Sumathipala *et al.*, 2000). The key lies in not dismissing the complaint because it has no somatic basis, but in recognising that mental illness is as much a health problem with specific interventions. The extended implication is the recognition that social problems such as domestic violence can be associated with a gynaecological complaint through the mediating influence of mental distress.

Perhaps the greatest policy implication, however, would be to force us to reconsider the categorical paradigms of health which continue to govern research designs and clinical services. Even though reproductive health has been defined as a 'state of complete physical, mental and social well-being' by the World Health Organisation, the reality is that mental health is still very much of peripheral concern both in research and in programme development. Women's health needs increasingly involve problems beyond reproduction, and it is our contention that mental health already is and will continue to grow to become a core health issue for women. The intersection of reproductive health and mental health provides an avenue for exploring these issues using already existing networks and resources and without risking the stigmatisation of women who would, otherwise, not wish to be associated with a 'mental illness'. While it may be premature to suggest interventions that address mental health issues, reproductive health researchers should take the initiative to provide sufficient evidence to policy-makers and health programmers that mental health matters too.

## REFERENCES


Agarwal, P., Malik, S. and Padubidri, V. (1990): 'A Study of Psychiatric Morbidity in a Gynaecology Outpatient Clinic', *Indian Journal of Psychiatry;* 32: 57-63

Bang, R, and Bang, A. (1996): 'Women's Perceptions of White Vaginal Discharge: Ethnographic Data from Rural Maharashtra' in Gittelsohn J., Bentley M.E., Pelto, P.J., Nag, M., Pachauri, S., Harrison, A. *et al.*, (eds), *Listening to Women Talk about their Health: Issues and Evidence from India.* New Delhi: Ford Foundation, 79-94.

Blue, I., Ducci, M.E., Jaswal, S., Ludermir, A. and Harpham, T. (1995): 'The Mental Health of Low-Income Urban Women: Case Studies From Bombay, India; Olinda, Brazil; and Santiago,Chile' in Harpham, T., Blue, T., (eds) *Urbanization and Mental Health in Developing Countries.* Aldershot: Avebury: 75-101.

Chaturvedi, S., Chandra, P., Isaac, M.K. and Sudarshan, C. (1993): 'Somatization Misattributed to Non-Pathological Vaginal Discharge', *Journal of Psychosomatic Research:* 17: 575-579.

Chaturvedi, S. (1988): 'Psychaesthenic Syndrome Related to Leukorrhea in Indian Women', *Journal of Psychosomatic Obstetrics and Gynecology:* 8: 67-72.

Davar, B. (1999): *The Mental Health of Indian Women: A Feminist Agenda.* New Delhi: Sage (India).

Ford Foundation (1997): Advocacy for Reproductive Health and Women's Empowerment in India, New Delhi.

Gath, D., Osborn, M., Bungay, G., Iles, S., Day, A., Bond, A. *et al.*, (1987): 'Psychiatric Disorder and Gynaecological Symptoms in Middle Aged Women: A Community Survey', *British Medical Journal:* 144: 28-34.

Goldberg, D. and Huxley, P. (1992): *Common Mental Disorders: A Bio-social Model.* London: Tavistock/Routledge.

Hawkes, S., Morison, L., Foster, S., Gausia, K., Chakraborty, J., Peeling, R.W. *et al.*, (1999): 'Managing Reproductive Tract Infections in Women in Low-Income, Low-Prevalence Situations: An Evaluation of Syndromic Management in Matlab, Bangladesh', *Lancet:* 354: 1776-1781.

Hodgkiss, A.D., Sufraz, R. and Watson, J.P. (1994): 'Psychiatric Morbidity and Illness Behaviour in Women with Chronic Pelvic Pain', *Journal of Psychosomatic Research:* 38: 3-9

Hotopf, M., Mayou, R., Wadsworth, M. and Wessely, S. (1998): 'Temporal Relationship Between Physical Symptoms and Psychiatric Disorder', *British Journal of Psychiatry:* 173: 255-261.

Hunter, M. (1990): 'Gynaecological Complaints' in Bass C (ed), *Somatization: Physical Symptoms and Psychological Illness*. Oxford: Blackwell Scientific Press: 235-258.

International Institute for Population Sciences and ORC Macro (2001): *National Family Health Survey-2, 1998-99:* India, Mumbai.

IUSSP Committee on Reproductive Health and University of Wistwaterand, (1997): *Gender, Reproductive Health and Weakness: Experiences of Slum Dwelling Women in Bombay, India.* 97: South Africa: Rustenburg.

Katon, W. and Walker, E.A. (1998): 'Medically Unexplained Symptoms in Primary Care', *Journal of Clinical Psychiatry*: 59 (suppl 20): 15-21.

Koenig, M., Jejeebhoy, S., Singh, S. and Sridhar, S. (1998): 'Investigating Women's Gynaecological Morbidity in India: Not just Another KAP Survey', *Reproductive Health Matters:* 6: 1-13.

Linden, M., Lecrubier, Y., Bellantuono, C., Benkert, O., Kisely, S. and Simon, G. (1999): 'The Prescribing of Psychotropic Drugs by Primary Care Physicians: An International Collaborative Study', *Journal of Clinical Psychopharmacology:* 19: 132-140.

Malhotra, H.K. and Wig, N.N. (1975): 'Dhat Syndrome: A Culture-Bound Sex Neurosis of the Orient'. *Archives of Sexual Medicine:* 4: 519-528.

Mumford, D.B. (1993): 'Somatization: A Transcultural Perspective', *International Review of Psychiatry:* 5: 231-242.

Murray, C. and Lopez, A. (1996): *The Global Burden of Disease*. Boston: Harvard School of Public Health, WHO and World Bank.

Ormel, J., Von Korff, M., Ustun, T.B., Pini, S., Korten, A. and Oldehinkel, T. (1994): 'Common Mental Disorders and Disability Across Cultures. *JAMA:* 272: 1741-1748.

Patel, V., Pereira, J. and Mann, A. (1998): 'Somatic and Psychological Models of Common Mental Disorders in India', *Psychological Medicine:* 28: 135-143.

Patel, V., Pereira, J., Coutinho, L., Fernandes, R., Fernandes, J. and Mann, A. (1998): 'Poverty, Psychological Disorder and Disability in Primary Care Attenders in Goa, India', *British Journal of Psychiatry:* 171: 533-536.

Patel, V., Araya, R., Lima, M.S., Ludermir, A. and Todd, C. (1999): 'Women, Poverty and Common Mental Disorders in Four Restructuring Societies', *Social Science and Medicine:* 49: 1461-1471.

Patel, V., Abas, M., Broadhead, J., Todd, C. and Reeler, A.P. (2001): 'Depression in Developing Countries: Lessons from Zimbabwe', *British Medical Journal.*

Pearce, S. and Beard, R.W. (1990): 'Chronic Pelvic Pain in Women' in: Bass C. (ed), *Somatization: Physical Symptoms And Psychological Illness*, Oxford: Blackwell Scientific Press: 259-275.

Patel, V., Chisholm, D., Rabe-Hesketh, S., Dias-Saxena, F., Andrew, G. and Mann, A. (in press): 'The Efficacy and Cost-Effectiveness of a Drug and Psychological Treatment for Common Mental Disorders in General Health Care in Goa, India: A Randomised Controlled Trial', *Lancet*.

Sumathipala, A., Hewege, S., Hanwella, R. and Mann, H. (2000): 'Randomized Controlled Trial of Cognitive Behaviour Therapy for Repeated Consultations for Medically Unexplained Complaints: A Feasibility Study in Sri Lanka', *Psychological Medicine:* 30: 747-757.

Tanksale, V., Sahasrabhojanee, M., Patel, V., Nevrekar, P., Menezes, S. and Mabey, D. (in press): 'The Reliability of a Structured Examination Protocol and Self-Administered Vaginal Swabs: A Pilot Study of Gynaecological Out-Patients in Goa, India', *Sexually Transmitted Infections*.

World Health Organization (1995): *The World Health Report 1995: Bridging the Gaps. Geneva:* World Health Organization.

# 6

# PROMOTING THE POSITIVE

## Maternal Mental Health and Child Development

*Nandita de Souza and Marcus Hughes*

There are several important reasons why women's mental health should receive special attention from health policy-makers and researchers. The strongest argument is that women are at particular risk of developing depression, which has been acknowledged by the World Health Organisation as the fourth leading cause of disability world-wide, and is predicted to rise to be the second leading cause by the year 2020 (WHO website). Furthermore, the excess of psychological distress falling on women appears not to be simply an artefact resulting from western-biased diagnostic systems. When women's mental health is examined from an anthropological perspective, without pre-conceived notions of diagnostic categories, the conclusions are the same. Studies from regions as widely-spread as South America, the Mediterranean, and Asia have identified locally-distinct idioms for psychological distress, and have consistently shown higher prevalence in women than men (Desjarlais *et al.*, 1995).

Although depression is significantly more common in women than in men, and problems of drug and alcohol misuse are more common in men, it is generally the case that all psychiatric conditions affect both men and women. In one particular case however, women's mental health is deserving of special attention because a group of psychological disturbances are exclusive to women. These are the psychological conditions related to pregnancy and childbirth, and they consist of antenatal anxiety and depression, the post-partum blues ('baby blues'), puerperal psychosis, and post-natal or post-partum depression. There is little or no research information relating to either the post-partum blues or puerperal psychosis from any low income country, so these conditions will not be considered further in this paper. Instead, we will focus on antenatal anxiety and depression, and post-natal depression (PND) as conditions under active investigation in Goa, as well as other parts of the world.

## Puerperal Mental Illness in Context

Psychiatric researchers and clinicians have not yet reached a final understanding of the interaction between a woman's mental state and childbearing. The traditional view, held from the 1960s until the 1990s, was to see pregnancy as a time of psychological stability, with a watershed at the time of delivery, after which women were prone to various degrees of psychological distress over and above their usual susceptibility. It was believed that this additional burden of puerperal mental disorder might persist for six months to a year after childbirth.

Several persuasive pieces of research, from both high and low income countries have challenged the orthodoxy presented above. One of these studies was conducted in Goa, and is discussed in detail later in this paper. The emerging conclusion of the newer research into maternal mental health is that the previous understanding was an over-simplification. It is now clear that psychological symptoms are common during pregnancy, and that the post-natal period is not a time of particularly raised risk of depression for women. However, we will argue that the diagnosis of PND is still an important one, not because more women are depressed after childbirth, but because depression after childbirth is more serious than at other times.

In addition to clarifying the time-course of psychological symptoms related to childbirth, medical research has succeeded in providing some clarification of the causes of post-natal depression. There is very little evidence that PND has a strong 'biological' component; contrary to the generally-held belief, it is unlikely that hormonal fluctuations in the post-natal period have a major role in causing PND. The most commonly-identified predisposing factors for PND are poor or unsupportive relationships, a past history of psychological disturbance, and psychological symptoms during pregnancy (O'Hara *et al.*, 1996). Therefore, the emerging 'medical model' of PND that will be adopted in this paper is of a common condition, with a predominantly psycho-social causation, and of importance primarily because the post-natal period is an especially bad time for a woman to be depressed.

However, before we settle on the use of psychiatric diagnostic terminology to discuss psychological distress related to childbirth, we will consider two important sources of dissent from the medical model—the anthropological critique, and the feminist critique.

## Anthropological Critiques of Post-natal Depression

Anthropologists have justifiably questioned the use of the diagnostic label of 'post-natal depression', originally claiming that ethnographic research from traditional societies indicated that PND may not be a universal phenomenon. A paper by Stern and Kruckman in 1983 reviewed the ethnographic research relating to events surrounding childbirth, in various ethnic groups around the world (Stern *et al.*, 1983). The authors found "surprisingly little evidence of the phenomenon identified in Western psychiatric diagnoses and in popular notions as post-partum depression." Their starting point was a study by Pillsbury, in which the post-natal routines among traditional Taiwan-Chinese women were examined (Pillsbury, 1978). Pillsbury discovered the near-universal practice of 'doing the month', in which a strict set of restrictions and privileges are applied to the newly-delivered mother for a full month. Although the primary focus of Pillsbury's account was the meaning of the practice itself, she noted

> This extra attention their families and social networks show them seems, in fact, to preclude Chinese women from experiencing post-partum depression as understood and so taken for granted by Americans.........Neither the Chinese translation of the term 'post-partum depression' nor the concept itself makes much sense to the majority of my informants.

Stern and Kruckman did not have a great deal more ethnographic data to support this as a general finding, but they did present a compelling account of the extensiveness of post-natal rituals, and more particularly the amount of extra support provided to new mothers in traditional agricultural societies. The hypothesis that these authors then proposed was that post-natal depression is unique to Western, industrialised societies, and that its causation lies in the loss of previously universal patterns of maternal support. Later in this paper, we will consider data from post-natal research in Goa, both anthropological and epidemiological, which challenges the view that PND is a phenomenon unique to western, industrialised societies. But the anthropological literature does raise the interesting question of the relationship between loss of traditional support structures and PND, and therefore how the prevalence of PND can be expected to change in societies 'in transition', of which Goa is clearly an example. Furthermore, the extension of the Stern and Kruckman hypothesis is that provision of extra support to a newly-delivered mother may alleviate PND. There is strong evidence from Western studies that simple, individual support can reduce the prevalence of PND, and we will describe later in this paper how similar approaches are being attempted under research conditions in Goa.

### The Feminist Perspective

One feminist writer, Oakley, has objected vehemently to the use of the term post-natal depression, stating "Science, responding to an agenda of basically social concerns, has provided the label 'post-natal depression' as a pseudo scientific tag for the description and ideological transformation of maternal discontent" (Oakley, 1980). However, there is plenty of evidence from the Western media that the label of PND, far from being foisted on women, is welcomed as a recognition of psychological distress that had traditionally been unacknowledged. A descriptive study of mothers in 1983 identified unexpected emotional stresses, arising from "the effort, work and disruption to life that parenthood and dependency brought with it" (Moss *et al.,* 1988). Similarly, qualitative research from Goa indicates that at least some women do recognise that distressing psychological symptoms can arise in the post-natal period (Rodrigues, 2002). Therefore the hard-line feminist approach taken by Oakley appears to lack general support from women themselves, and women seem more ready to align themselves with a medical model of PND.

Another social scientist, Steinberg, offers an approach to PND which preserves the consideration of the political economy in the illness of PND, without detracting from the distressing experiences of women. "The previous emphasis has been upon [..] fascinating descriptions of rites and rituals......Currently, social and health problems are addressed as: poverty, gender issues, marital disruption, unjustified use of medical interventions, domestic violence and dislocation of refugees" (Steinberg, 1996). We propose that the medical model of PND is useful in identifying distress on an individual level, and allowing resources to be allocated to help relieve this distress. The resources may be from within the family, such as reducing the load of household chores placed on a newly-delivered mother. But the resources may also offered from within medical services, if appropriate forms of psycho-social intervention can be developed for PND.

What the medical community can learn from feminist contributions to the literature is to see PND in its wider social context; as a condition with an important element of social causation, and at its worst as a diagnostic label imposed by a clinician without regard to whether the woman herself feels in need of assistance.

## Maternal Mental Illness in Goa and Beyond

### *The Goa Depression After Childbirth Study*

It is reasonable to question how important a problem post-natal depression is for Goan women. To answer this, there are precise and comprehensive data available from the Depression After Childbirth study (DAC study), the results of which have recently been published in a major psychiatric journal (Patel *et al.*, 2002). The striking findings of this research were that 23 per cent of childbearing women fulfilled criteria for post-natal depression when interviewed six weeks after delivery. This prevalence of PND is high compared to the rates found among women in Europe and USA, where a meta-analysis has estimated the prevalence of PND to be 13 per cent. However, a study from a township in South Africa has detected a much higher prevalence of PND at 34.7% in a population suffering extreme economic and social deprivation (Cooper *et al.*, 1999). Therefore rates of PND in Goan women appear to be high compared to Western women, but lower than the prevalence in at least one very low income non-Western population.

## Goan Women's Explanatory Models for PND

The investigators in the DAC study recognised that the diagnostic construct of PND may be an alien one among Goan women, so alongside the epidemiological cohort study, they also completed a qualitative research component (Rogrigues, 2002). They used individual in-depth interviews with a group of depressed women, as well as a group of non-depressed women, and some of their husbands. The investigators explored the explanatory models used by Goan women to conceptualise psychological distress associated with childbirth, and assessed the extent of concordance with psychiatric diagnostic constructs. The results of this qualitative research have been submitted for publication, and they will provide the cultural context within which the results of the DAC study can be more fully understood.

### *The Pattern of Psychological Morbidity in Childbearing Women*

Data from the DAC study, which sampled women attending a hospital antenatal clinic, reveal that levels of psychological symptoms were high during pregnancy (Patel *et al.,* 2002). Thus 41.9 per cent of women scored 5 or more on the 12-item General Health Questionnaire (GHQ-12), indicating clinically significant psychological morbidity using a standard psychometric instrument. The investigators estimated that only 22 per cent of cases of 'post-natal' depression were new-onset cases in the post-natal period; the majority of post-natally depressed women had psychological symptoms during pregnancy too. Although the GHQ-12 is a different instrument from the Edinburgh Post-natal Depression Scale (EPDS) (Cox *et al.,* 1987) that was used to determine rates of PND post-natally, the DAC study does lend support to the growing consensus that psychological symptoms in pregnancy are as common, if not commoner, than in the post-natal period. This in turn has led to efforts to include psychological intervention in the antenatal care of at vulnerable women, on the basis that symptoms are often present during pregnancy, earlier intervention might be expected to be more effective, and pregnancy is a time of easier access to women, when they are in regular contact with health services. The Goa 'Supporting Mothers in Pregnancy Study (SMIPS)' described below is one such programme, offering a psycho-social supportive intervention to women both before and after childbirth to determine, among other outcomes of interest, whether rates of post-natal depression are reduced by such an intervention.

### *The Causes of Depression Among Childbearing Women*

By using a cohort study design, in which women were recruited and interviewed antenatally, and then re-interviewed and diagnosed post-natally, the DAC study investigators were able to identify the factors that are predictive of post-natal depression in Goan women (Patel *et al.,* 2002). Over 11 different antenatal variables were considered in the analysis, and over 12 different post-natal variables. When all the antenatal variables were adjusted for, those that remained significant predictors of PND were antenatal psychiatric morbidity (which increased the odds of PND by six times) and the current pregnancy being unplanned, which increased the odds by 3.3 times. When all the post-natal variables were considered in an adjusted analysis, those that remained significant were problems with breastfeeding, infant hospital admission, and sadness about the newborn baby's gender.

### *Infant Gender and Post-natal Depression*

The Goa DAC study was the first in the world to demonstrate that infant gender could be a risk factor for post-natal depression, albeit an indirect one. Although not a predictor of post-natal depression in its own right, it appears that delivering a female child functioned as an 'activator' for a number of other risk factors. Thus marital violence and hunger due to poverty were not risk factors in women delivering boys, but they were significant risk factors for post-natal depression in women delivering a girl. Similarly, unhappiness about the infant's gender, and already having a female child were predictive of depression only in women who delivered a girl child. The investigators pointed to the recognised pressures among Indian women to deliver at least one male child. We propose that the potential for strong gender bias to precipitate maternal mental illness in vulnerable women is entirely consistent with the recognised psycho-social causation of PND.

### *The Consequences of Maternal Mental Illness for the Mother Herself*

Depression in the post-natal period makes the already-difficult task of parenting a neonate even more arduous. Many women will be anaemic, marginally nourished, physically drained, overworked, sleep-deprived, and anxious about their new parenting responsibilities. Depression adds to these burdens, by making the sufferer feel exhausted on minimal effort, and have difficulty sleeping even when the opportunity presents itself. The DAC study showed that two-thirds of the women who are depressed at six weeks after delivery remain depressed until at least six months post-partum. At six months, depressed women were significantly disabled by their symptoms, in comparison to non-depressed women; they spent double the number of days unable to complete their daily activities, and required more medical attention.

Depressed women tend to think the worst of themselves, including their adequacy as parents, and usually find little rewarding or enjoyable in the experience. When depressed mothers present to health services, the problem is often framed as that of an inconsolable, crying baby, or as problems with breastfeeding. Indeed, when considering the higher rate of breastfeeding problems among depressed women in the DAC study, it is likely that at least some of these cases were women who were managing adequately, but were overly critical of their own performance, as a result of the depression. This problem is not trivial-unduly critical self-evaluation of breastfeeding may result in early discontinuation and substitution with commercial powdered 'formula' milk, with a loss of the advantages of breast over bottle feeding. The following section of this paper examines several other ways in which maternal depression can have serious consequences for her infant's development.

## The Effects of Maternal Depression on Child Development

Maternal mental health and child development are inextricably linked since the mother is most often the child's first and foremost carer. Research has amply proven this through several studies, which have explored the effects of post-natal depression on children at various ages. Not just the presence, but also the chronicity of maternal depression has an important impact on the child's health and development.

### *The Impact of Maternal Depression on Infant Growth and Development: Data from Goa*

Within the Goa 'Depression After Childbirth Study' described above, a further nested case control study was performed to compare the growth and development of babies of depressed and non-depressed mothers at the age of 6 months using standardized measures (Patel *et al.,* 2002). The results were unambiguous. Babies whose mothers were depressed had poorer growth and development outcomes. Although there is mounting evidence of child developmental problems resulting from maternal depression, this study provided the first indication that poor infant physical growth could be linked to maternal mental status. These results have considerable public health significance for a country like India, where early indications are that many women may suffer from post-natal depression, and multiple other factors operate to compromise child nutrition and development.

The work assessing the infant consequences of maternal depression is just beginning in Goa. However, research from Western countries has already well underway in demonstrating the range of infant developmental outcomes that may be affected by maternal mental illness. Key areas of this research are summarised below.

### *The Effects of Maternal Depression on Infant Social Development*

The social and emotional development of infants in this context has been studied in three ways *i.e.* maternal infant interactions, quality of infant attachment to the mother and presence of behaviour difficulties.

Detailed observations within the first three months after childbirth have provided fascinating information about the very early effects of maternal mood on the mother-infant relationship. Babies from disadvantaged families whose mothers were depressed showed more protest behaviour, withdrawal, avoidance, fussing and fewer positive facial expressions in their interactions with their mothers (Field *et al.,* 1988; Cohn *et al.,* 1986). However other studies which have assessed women from more socio-economically privileged classes have not shown any significant difference in the interactions between depressed and non-depressed mothers and their infants (Murray *et al.*, 1996a). Therefore it appears that there is a critical interplay of post-natal depression and social adversity on infant responses.

Studies of attachment to the mother, usually measured after the infant is 18 months old, have produced conflicting results (Murray *et al.*, 1996b). Insecure attachment, with the predominant pattern being one of avoidance has been found in later infancy in children of post-natally depressed mothers. However another study of mothers from a low-risk sample did not reveal any differences in the attachment quality of babies of depressed and non-depressed mothers. Behaviour difficulties in 18-month infants related to eating, sleeping, separation and temper tantrums were more likely to be reported by mothers who had suffered from PND. Independent assessment of the behaviour of pre-school children by their teachers showed that more anti-social behaviour was reported for boys of mothers who had been depressed.

### *The Effects of Maternal Depression on Infant Intellectual Development*

The effect of maternal mood disorder on the cognitive development of children is another area of prolific research. Poorer infant mental development, especially in boys has been reported (Murray, 1992). These impairments persist into childhood too, as two British studies have demonstrated (Sharp *et al.*, 1995; Cogill *et al.*, 1986). However, again the effects appear to be mediated through social adversity, as when a low-risk population was studied, there was no relationship between post-natal depression and cognitive development of 5 year old children ( Murray *et al.*, 1996c).

The question that is most pertinent is how these effects occur. There appear to be 3 mechanisms.

1. The direct impact of the exposure of the child to maternal depressive symptoms.
2. The altered interaction between the depressed mother and baby.

3. The added effect of environmental variables such as social adversity, which occur with depression.

Considering that some women may be depressed for a few weeks, and others for several months, the question arises as to whether the later child effects of PND require the depression to be chronic. In the case of both socialisation problems and cognitive under-performance, the answer appears to be that adverse effects can continue to accrue, even after the maternal depression has subsided. This raises the possibility that 'sensitive periods' might exist in a child's developmental timetable, during which he or she is specifically sensitive to wrong cues. It appears that post-natal depression, which has its peak prevalence between 6 and 12 weeks post-partum, may be prone to occur at just such a sensitive time in childhood social development.

In summary, findings from research both in Goa and elsewhere are beginning to piece together a complicated picture in which there is no doubt that post-natal depression can have lasting adverse consequences for the newly-delivered infant, particularly in the presence of social adversity. These findings, together, with the impact of PND on the mother and family, add considerable weight to the argument for considering PND to be a public health priority.

## Other Influences on Child Development

Post-natal depression is not the only parental psychological factor of importance in child development; there are other influences of the wider psycho-social environment within the household. Here, we consider neonates who are at increased risk of developmental delay for physical reasons, particularly those whose condition is compromised at birth, by very low birthweight, breathing problems, seizures, etc. Although these neonatal problems affect all social groups, they are commoner in circumstances of psycho-social deprivation, where antenatal care, maternal nutrition and facilities for delivery may have been less than ideal. The immediate medical needs of the neonate are often paramount in such cases, and many of these babies will be admitted to a neonatal intensive care unit, if available. Once the immediate medical crisis has passed, and the neonate is discharged from hospital, the home environment becomes an important determinant of the infant's developmental trajectory. Here, parental capacity, and in particular the environment created by the baby's mother, can significantly influence the developmental outcome for her child. A developmentally optimal environment includes physical and emotional security, and regular displays of affection by the parents, as well as stimulation across different sensory modalities-particularly auditory, visual and tactile. The nutrition of the baby is as important as its physical environment, and research shows that maintenance of breastfeeding is another important means of improving infant developmental outcomes.

For various reasons, parents often miss opportunities to optimise the environment in which their infant is developing— for example, parents may be unaware of the importance of providing for their baby in these ways, or they may be overworked, stressed, pre-occupied, or under-confident in their role as parents and agents in their infant's development. The majority of infants may be able to survive sub-optimal rearing environments without undue effects on their developmental progress, but 'high risk' neonates, such as those admitted to neonatal intensive care units deserve special support in providing an improved rearing environment. Some simple 'early intervention' approaches have been developed to allow parents to enrich the developmental environment in the infant's household; these include early infant stimulation exercises for visual, auditory and tactile sensory modalities, as well as the active support of breastfeeding. The application of these approaches in the Sangath-CRY early intervention programme is described below.

In the following section of this paper, we describe five projects that have been, or are being conducted in Goa, to intervene with mothers and their babies to promote positive maternal and child mental health, drawing on some of the priorities that have been identified in the research evidence.

## Promoting the Positive: Interventions for Maternal and Child Mental Health

### *Extending Antenatal Care*

Having demonstrated the close associations between maternal mental health and child health, our focus should be on what we can do to enhance both. It is clear that we must start in the antenatal period itself. For most childbearing women in Goa, formal antenatal care is restricted to brief obstetric check-ups, yet there are excellent and affordable models from overseas where midwives offer antenatal classes to capitalise on an opportunity for health promotion. Such antenatal classes can provide much-needed education concerning maternal nutrition and early identification of obstetric problems, together with baby care and promotion of breastfeeding. With a national prevalence of 30 per cent low birth weight in India, prevention of malnutrition seems to be a priority, and an educational approach is likely to be more sustainable than providing food handouts, even if the latter has been shown to improve birth weights. Antenatal classes that provide not just health education and pregnancy advice, but also render emotional support that can greatly enhance the mental and reproductive health of mothers. Baby Talk, at Sangath is an example of an antenatal class initiative provided as a service in North Goa. Though we do not have any research data to present, the acceptance of the Baby Talk programme and the positive feedback we have received informs us that such support is valuable. In our research programme, antenatal education is an important component of the intervention in the SMIP study, described below.

## Prevention of Post-natal Depression and Its Effects

### *Supporting Mothers in Pregnancy Study (SMIPS)*

The hypothesis of the SMIP study is that certain women might benefit from additional support in the last few weeks of pregnancy and the early weeks after delivery. This hypothesis is being tested by means of a randomised, controlled clinical trial, in which 380 volunteer pregnant women will eventually participate. Half the women will receive a supportive intervention, and the other half will receive their usual care from obstetric and medical services. The research intervention consists of a home-based programme of psycho-social support, provided by a community support worker. The programme consists of five or six sessions, two antenatally in the last two months of pregnancy, and three or four post-natally, until ten weeks postpartum. The antenatal sessions include a large component of education and preparation for childbirth, together with supportive challenging of gender bias. The post-natal sessions are more individualised, to provide support specific to the needs of the woman herself, but they also include elements of breastfeeding support, and infant stimulation and massage. The intervention programme was designed following focus group discussions with newly-delivered Goan mothers, consultation with experienced community practitioners, analysis of the research literature, and a pilot study in Goa with 20 women, which included detailed feedback on the programme.

The study will determine outcomes in four domains, comparing control and intervention groups, at both 3 and 6 months post-partum. Maternal mental health will be assessed using standard diagnostic instruments to determine the prevalence of post-natal depression, as well as associated disability symptoms. Infant development will be assessed by measuring growth, as well as a detailed developmental assessment at 6 months. The quality of the mother-infant relationship will be assessed at 3 months by micro-analysis of video-taped interactions in standardised situations. Finally, an economic analysis will be made of costs of healthcare for mother and child in the post-partum period.

### *The Secondary Prevention of Developmental Disorders in High Risk Neonates*

#### *The Sangath-CRY Early Intervention Programme*

We know that maternal health and infant health are closely related. Therefore any threat to the child's well-being is going to affect the mother too. Parents of babies at high-risk for development and growth problems often feel overwhelmed and helpless in the face of innumerable care issues ranging from breastfeeding to infant stimulation to immunization. Family building through the provision of support to mothers and fathers is vital. This was the focus of the Sangath-CRY early intervention programme, where a team of health professionals, as well as trained Anganwadi workers guided parents in their daily travails of caring for a vulnerable infant. Parents were encouraged to think of themselves as trainers of their babies. Mothers were provided advice on feeding, stimulation, child development and common behaviour problems, giving emphasis to strategies that could be used within the home, relying on resources that were readily available to them. Anganwadi workers from Bicholim taluka were also trained to provide this support. Community involvement through the Mahila Swasthya Samitis was strengthened by having regular discussions related to child growth, development and nutrition with women of child-bearing age. Thus a network of maternal support systems can be energised within the community.

### *Promotion and Support of Breastfeeding*

#### *Mothers Understand Mothers (MUMs) Programme*

*MUMs:* Breastfeeding difficulties can be rather acute and worrisome to mothers as they struggle through the early days of parenting. Since nutrition is so closely tied to nurturing in India, lactation failure is often viewed as bad mothering. Anxiety related to feeding only adds to the mother's emotional burden. Therefore providing adequate support to the mother during the initiation and establishment of breastfeeding will have a major impact on how she faces the challenges of mothering. This is what MUMs (Mothers Understand Mothers) seeks to do. It is a collective of mothers and trained lactation experts who provide advice and support for breastfeeding difficulties to mothers in the post-natal period, through direct or telephonic contact. These "experts" are "confidence tricksters" in actual fact, as they use their training and own successful breastfeeding experiences to convince new mothers to show the world what breasts are for!

### *Clinical Services for Children and their Families*

#### *The Sangath Child Development Clinic*

*Support of mothers:* Mothers often accompany the children who are brought to the Child Development Centre at Sangath. They are the ones who worry the most and often blame themselves for their child's difficulties. There is much that can be achieved by strengthening and encouraging what the mother is doing correctly—which is often a lot. The child is the entrance to the mother's world, as women are often averse to seeking help for their own difficulties. Somehow, consulting the helping professional "for the sake of the child" is a legitimate action. However if we neglect to address the mother's personal issues and concerns, both assessment and therapy of the child's problems are likely to fail.

*Parenting:* "Parenting" is a catchword that has become a fashionable concept for modern-day, urban families. It is common knowledge that the way in which a child is brought up in the home has a significant influence on his or her eventual outcome, be it in the emotional, academic or occupational areas. The Sangath Centre conducts a wide variety of workshops designed to assist parents with the day-to-day demands of raising children. The primary aim of the Centre is to prevent behavioural and emotional problems in children by enhancing the skills and confidence of parents and by addressing the family risk factors known to contribute to adverse developmental outcomes in children.

Information materials designed for parents are also provided to deal with problem behaviours, and to prevent more severe behaviour problems from arising. Therapist contact is intended to support parents in using positive parenting strategies involving a combination of instructions, modelling, marital communication skills and stress coping skills.

## The Future—Community-based Surveillance and Interventions for Maternal and Child Health

Our detailed recommendations for developing maternal and child mental health care must await the outcome of the research projects currently underway. However, it is already clear that the potential exists to develop the community-based facilities for detection and intervention in maternal and child mental health. The optimistic scenario is that simple screening protocols will be developed to allow 'at-risk' individuals (both mother and child) to be identified; that by early identification of problems, simple intervention strategies can be used effectively; and that the burden of maternal and child mental health problems can be reduced by means of a cost-effective, community-based set of programmes.

The Anganwadi Worker (AW) holds the key to the health futures of the community. These grassroots workers command the respect and consideration of the populations they serve and are placed in a prime position to be harbingers of change in the health of mothers and children. Training the AW in maternal mental health and child development, especially the early detection of problems is crucial if the findings of research are to be translated into effective action in the community. Building the skills of the anganwadi worker in a range of supportive interventions for the mother and child creates a community resource that is available, acceptable and sustainable. The AW can also be trained to refer cases that require further assessment and more complex management as well as provide information to families of the availability of special schemes for persons with special needs. However, if Anganwadi workers are to take on a greater role as maternal and child health workers, it is essential for them to have appropriate support to do so. After initial training, they should be given refresher courses at regular intervals. Appropriate support systems must also be in place; there must be an agreed referral system by which cases of concern may be referred into the primary or secondary health services. And there must also be monitoring systems within the Integrated Child

Development Service, to ensure that the enhanced Anganwadi worker role is achieving its aims.

*Breast-feeding:* The simple strategy of promoting breastfeeding can have enormous impact on fostering child development. Breast milk has the vital ingredients for optimal brain growth and the closeness of the mother and baby at the time of feeding encourages bonding. Breast milk can prevent a horde of illnesses that can impair a child's growth and development. The breastfeeding movement can gain momentum through enlisting the help of other mothers who have had successful lactation experiences. As women reach out to support each other, their mutual empowerment can only be good for their wellness.

Parenting programmes to empower mothers and fathers in their care-giving can also impart skills that are vital in daily life. As mothers feel more competent in their care-giving role, their increased self-esteem and confidence will promote resilience to threats to their mental health.

## Conclusions

The indications from the research evidence are that the mental health of mothers requires some special consideration from health policy-makers, particularly with regard to the interaction between maternal and child mental health. Failure to address maternal and infant mental health problems can have serious consequences for both the mother herself and the developing child. Fortunately, increasing recognition of these problems and relationships has led to the development of intervention strategies to support mothers and their children. Several such intervention programmes have been initiated in Goa, some as health services, and others as research projects. While the research evidence for interventions is being established, it is likely that simple, culturally-appropriate measures will be the most practical approaches to improving maternal mental health. Such measures include developing the role of the Anganwadi worker to identify, and where possible support 'at risk' mothers and their babies.

**REFERENCES**

Cogill, S., Caplan, H., Alexandra, H. *et al.*, (1986): 'Impact of Post-natal Depression on Cognitive Development in Young Children', *British Medical Journal:* 292:1165-7.

Cohn, J., Matias, R., Tronick, E. *et al.*, (1986): 'Face-to-Face Interactions of Depressed Mothers and Their Infants'in Tronick E and Field T (eds), *Maternal Depression and Infant Disturbance (New Directions for Child Development, No. 34)*, San Francisco: Jossey-Bass.

Cooper, P.J., Tomlinson, M., Swartz, L., Woolgar, M., Murray, L. and Molteno, C. (1999): 'Post-partum Depression and the Mother-Infant Relationship in a South African Peri-Urban Settlement', *British Journal of Psychiatry:* 175:554-8.

Cox, J.L., Holden, J.M. and Sagovsky, R. (1987): 'Detection of Post-natal Depression. Development of the 10-item Edinburgh Post-natal Depression Scale', *British Journal of Psychiatry:* 150:782-6.

Desjarlais, R., Eisenberg, L., Good, B. and Kleinman, A. (eds) (1995): 'Women' in *World Mental Health. Problems and Priorities in Low Income Countries*, 179-206. New York, Oxford University Press.

Field, T., Healy, B., Goldstein, S., Perry, S. *et al.*, (1988): 'Infants of Depressed Mothers Show "Depressed" Behaviour Even with Non-depressed Adults', *Child Development :* 59:1569-79.

Moss, P. *et al.*, quoted in Elliott, S. *et al.*, (1988): 'Parents Groups in Pregnancy: A Preventative Intervention for Postnatal Depression?', in Gottleib (ed), *Marshaling Social Support*, Sage, California.

Murray, L., Fiori-Cowley, A., Hooper, R. (1996): 'The Impact of Post-natal Depression and Associated Adversity on Early Mother Infant Interactions and Later Infant Outcome', *Child Development:* 67:2512 26.

Murray, L. and Cooper, P. J. (1996): 'The Impact of Post-partum Depression on Child Development', *International Review of Psychiatry:* 8:55-63.

Murray, L. (1992): 'The Impact of Postnatal Depression on Infant Development', *Journal of Child Psychology and Psychiatry:* 33:543-61.

Murray, L., Hipwell, A., Hooper, R. *et al.*, (1996): 'The Cognitive Development of Five Year Old Children of Postnatally Depressed Mothers', *Journal of Child Psychology and Psychiatry:* 37:927-36.

O'Hara, M.W. and Swain, A.M. (1996): 'Rates and Risk of Post-partum Depression: A Meta-Analysis', *International Review of Psychiatry:* 8: 37-54.

Oakley, A. (1980): *Women Confined*, Oxford: Martin Robertson.

Patel, V., De Souza, N., and Rodrigues, M., 'Post-natal Depression and Infant Growth and Development in Low-Income Countries: A Cohort Study From Goa, India'. *(Personal Communication).*

Patel, V., Rodrigues, M. and De Souza, N. (2002): 'Gender, Poverty and Postnatal Depression: A Cohort Study from Goa, India', *American Journal of Psychiatry*: 159: 43-7.

Pillsbury, B. (1978): "Doing the Month': Confinement and Convalescence of Chinese Women after Childbirth', *Social Science and Medicine*: 12: 11-22.

Rodrigues, M. 2002. *(Personal Communication).*

Steinberg, S. (1996): 'Childbearing Research: A Transcultural Review', *Social Science and Medicine*: 43:1765-84.

Stern, G. and Kruckman, L. (1983): 'Multi-Disciplinary Perspectives on Post-partum Depression: An Anthropological Critique', *Social Science and Medicine*: 17:1027-41.

Sharp, D., Hay, D., Pawlby, S. *et al.*, (1995): 'The Impact of Post-natal Depression on Boys' Intellectual Development', *Journal of Child Psychology and Psychiatry*: 36:1315-36.

WHO website, Brundtland, Harlem G., Director-General of WHO. 'Global Perspectives on Mental Health': 15-9-2000.

# 7

# A TREATMENT FOR COMMON MENTAL DISORDERS IN THE COMMUNITY

*Fiona Dias Saxena*

Health is defined differently by different sections of population. It may be viewed as a concept, a process or a goal. Health is influenced by many factors that interact which each other. When the interaction is positive it brings about health, otherwise one suffers from illness. The factors that influence health are biological, behavioural, socio-economical, political and environmental. Biological influences are those such as sex, race and nutrition and developmental changes. The behavioural include those that are consciously or unconsciously learned in the home, school or in the cultural milieu. The socio-economic factors are those that are related to social status, life style and others. Political factors relate to power, will, your ability to make decisions, the ability one has to influence others. Environment includes the physical, psychological and social milieu that can help or hinder health.

## Background

In 1998, Sangath Centre conducted a study titled 'Treatment of Depression' in 2 public health hospitals, namely the Asilo and Hospicio in North and South Goa. The study was to find out whether counselling or medication or a combination of both work in the treatment of common mental disorders. The subjects were selected randomly from the OPD of the hospital and were administered a General Health Questionnaire comprising of 12 questions. If they scored above 7 on this then with their compliance they were administered the CISR - a standardised questionnaire validated in Konkani to check depression. Only those who scored high and were depressed were sent for counselling or medication/placebo.

Of the sample, 150 cases were found to have mild or moderate depression and were sent for counselling. Eighty-four of them were women and of these 35 had suffered from family violence, which was the primary cause of their depression. Their symptoms were sleep disorders, lack of appetite, headaches, dizziness, aches and pains, palpitations. On closer inquiry, some had suicidal thoughts, low self-esteem, feelings of anxiety and numbness etc.

Counselling using the problem solving approach was used with those who were willing and compliant. This involved using whatever community resources were available, resources available from the government, support from family and friends, networking with allied systems, legal aid cells, women's groups and child care centres.

Since the population was semi-literate to totally non-reading, one had to use charts and anecdotes while counselling. Incidentally, if the client needed to be assertive in some situations, role-play was used much to the initial amusement of the clients. The population that interested me, were women as men were not too compliant either because the counsellor was a woman, or because they favoured medication to counselling. Amongst the women, the 33 per cent of women who were victims of family violence were followed up, through letters or messages sent to monitor their situations more closely.

Counselling played a significant role to help them get better. Medication, prescribed at the OPD, helped them feel better for a short time. Sleeping tablets did work for a short time. But their overall health did not improve and they would come again and again for treatment. Counselling in health care addresses not just the physical but also the social and the psychological and enhances the client to think of solutions and changes that need to be undertaken if better health is the aim. Counselling should be part of the health care system.

There were some limitations, which could be overcome if this facility was available at the Primary Health Centre. Travelling all the way to the hospital was not feasible and was expensive. Patients would feel more comfortable in their own milieu. In the case of depression due to family violence, patients said that their partners would be under greater social pressure if he/she were sent for by a health worker or counsellor to have a dialogue about his/her behaviour. Also the health worker could conduct a home visit to see the non-compliant clients and find out if there is something that needs to be addressed more seriously.

**Brief Profile of the Patients of the Treatment of Depression Study**

- Almost 70 per cent of the patients seen were women ranging between the age groups of 35 years of age to 70 years of age.
- All the patients belong to the lower socio-economic strata of society. They are engaged in subsistence farming and sometimes employed in other people's farms. Approximately on an average they earned about Rs. 40 to 60 per day. They use these earnings for daily household expenses and have neither savings nor any money kept aside for emergency.
- They all come from large families and have 3 to 5 children. Their village/community support systems are strong and they can seek help when they are in trouble.
- Very few of them knew to read and write, but have experienced a lot of hard times and have managed well through sheer common sense and resilience.
- Health related; they suffer from headaches, dizziness, aches and pains, heart diseases, low BP, anaemia and related problems.

Their main problems are related to growing unemployment, financial constraints and violence in the family due to alcoholism.

## Nirmaan—Building Sustainable Intervention in the Area of Family Violence

The lessons learnt from this study propelled the author to address depression of women with violence as a high risk factor through an intervention programme in the Sangath Centre. A fellowship was awarded by the Mac Arthur foundation for a programme entitled '*Nirmaan* (working with family violence)'. *Nirmaan* means to construct and implies building/rebuilding, which was the aim of the programme—either to rebuild a broken family, failing which to assist the individuals to rebuild their own lives and harmony.

The programme was conducted at the Sangath Centre. The Sangath Society is the leading provider of a multidisciplinary service for children, adolescents and families where women hold an important part. The clinical team comprises of a developmental paediatrician, a psychiatrist and epidemiologist, clinical psychologists, remedial teachers and social workers. Treatment is provided at the Centre and within the communities.

The programme tried to address intimate hurtful information by providing a safe space to talk about the trauma, to instil a process of trust over a period of time in the client no matter what ever happens and to counsel and assist the client psychologically to move on.

There were 3 main components of the programme

*Counselling:* Checking whether the index client is depressed and counselling both the client and the abuser. Also referring the children and teenagers for counselling.

*Advocacy and Networking:* There were a series of workshops for barefoot counsellors, street plays, having a dialogue and collaborating with Family Counselling services, Women 's organisations, Community/Village organisations, village priests and working with the allied systems like the police, a few medical personnel and legal personnel.

*Research:* Conducting a descriptive study on compliant women survivors of family violence undergoing common mental disorders and monitoring the intervention used.

**Research Methodology**

*Focus Group Discussions* – with recovered clients and some representatives of village groups and barefoot counsellors

*Development of an Interview Guide* – The guide was tested on 20 clients and then reviewed by experts like Dr. Surinder Jaswal (Tata Institute of Social Science) to check and comment on the same. Information was also sought from the faculty of Family Psychiatry Unit, NIMHAS, Bangalore. An interview guide was framed in English and later translated into Konkani through the back translation method.

The main themes that were discussed in the guide were:

- Information on socio-demographic details.
- What is the impact of violence on the social and economic status of the family?
- Description of the nature and form that violence takes. Is there a particular pattern?
- What is the cause as perceived by them?
- What is the mental state of the survivor?
- Are there any safety measures taken?
- How did the family and community respond to violence?
- Did they seek help, from whom and did they get it?
- Did they seek medical help?
- How did they overcome the violent situation?
- If they separated from the violator, what was the societal response?

*Interviewing Method:* The interview guide was used for 90 clients who were survivors of family violence; 89 of those interviewed were married. One was in a long-term relationship. The questions were asked in an open-ended fashion. A specific order of questioning was not followed; the women were allowed to talk sequentially based on the themes of the guide. Concrete examples were probed whenever necessary. They were allowed space for silence and expression of sadness. Survivors were also asked to invite anyone they were comfortable with to sit with them during the first interview if they desired. The recording was taken down verbatim. Most often the first interview was completed within an hour, but sometimes it was continued for another hour on another day.

*General Health Quotient (GHQ) Score:* This is a checklist of 12 questions that was checked and scored. If the client scores above 7 then one can suggest s/he is showing signs of mild or moderate depression.

## The Intervention

On completion of the interview guide we had a case conference and discussed the plan of action. The treatment would comprise of the 4 kinds of intervention, decided on a case-by-case basis and keeping in view the time frame the client is willing to spend on treatment. The treatment comprised of:

Individual Therapy
Family Therapy
Couple therapy.

Techniques used were Problem Solving, Cognitive and Behaviour Modifications, Supportive Techniques. The uniqueness of this programme was working with the perpetrator.

## Outcome Measures

The outcome measures used were:

1. To check whether violence had stopped or not through another short interview.
2. GHQ scores taken at the onset were compared to scores taken at the end of therapy, and after one year;
3. Qualitative information on what the women were doing 1 year after the intervention.

## Some of the Initial Findings with Regard to Counselling and Support

Women who attended more than five counselling sessions and took the treatment seriously did better than those who did not.

Their symptoms disappeared. Most of them used the problem solving approach. In some cases one had to use cognitive therapy as they had very low self-esteem and negative feelings about themselves. The use of drama and role-play were very useful in teaching survivors to be more assertive and confident. Many of them had phobias related to the violence experience and those were handled through exercises and planned activities. The survivors were allowed to bring in a good friend or confidante to the sessions if they desired.In almost all cases if the survivor's family was supportive they were consulted and encouraged to come for the sessions and continue supporting the survivors at home. Women who had family support did better than those who did not have this kind of support. If the women were placed temporarily in a shelter like Asha Bhavan in Goa, the superintendent of the shelter was in the know of the situation if the survivor allowed it and continues getting support and assistance to improve her situation and enable the depression to lift.

Women whose spouses (perpetrators) came for the sessions did better than those who did not. Unfortunately, only 33 spouses came for the sessions. Almost half of them reconciled while the remaining did not reconcile but were not antagonistic towards the survivor. They made amends for their behaviour and parted ways amicably, supporting the family with maintenance and followed a strict non-violent decorum when they came for visiting rights.

Those women, whose spouses did not comply, worked towards building their harmony with the support of family, friends and community. Many in this category moved out of the marriage and filed for judicial separation.

Most of the women did go to a General Practitioner, either privately or in a public hospital, some went to an orthopaedic and some went to a gynaecologist, a few visited a psychiatrist. They were given medication for their symptoms but the cause was not really addressed.

Counselling did assist in women making better and more focused decisions about their future and their relationship with the spouse. When one is depressed the decision taken at that time may not be the right one or that which the survivor really would desire.

## Significance of Advocacy snd Networking

Counselling coupled with advocacy helped the survivor to cope with the violence in the community. The street plays done in the villages where the target population came from and the workshops with barefoot counsellors from the same villages complemented the treatment. Besides this the networking with women's groups, the State Commission for Women and the police and the legal aid cell, when the perpetrator was not coming for a dialogue, and the village priests and community groups played a role towards easing the stress on the survivor and the subsequent depression that she underwent.

Very few survivors went to the police on their own. Some wanted legal advice but did not know where to go. This indicates that women have more access or rather are allowed to visit a doctor/hospital or health care facility when sick or bruised rather than a women's organisation or the police, hence it makes the health care system more responsible to attend and further refer her to an allied system for the welfare of her health and harmony.

The above findings have convinced the author that common mental disorder in women, with or without violence as a risk factor, can be treated at the level of the community. The Primary Health Centre can house a health worker who can be trained to be a barefoot counsellor, network with barefoot counsellors in the villages within the jurisdiction and attend to patients in the community. S/he can refer the patient appropriately and be referred to as a support agent. This will be explained in more detail in the latter part of the paper.

## Gender Violence and Health in Reproductive Years—An Issue to be Addressed

*Domestic/Family Violence* is the most common form of gender-based violence. In every country where reliable, large-scale studies on gender violence are available, upwards from 20 per cent of women have been abused by the men they live with. Abused women face a host of physical injuries that include chronic complaints such as headaches, abdominal pains, muscle aches, sleeping and eating disorders. Battered women are more likely to experience persistent miscarriages and recurrent vaginal infections. Fearful of using birth control, they are more likely to experience unwanted pregnancies and resort to illegal, unsafe abortions. Pregnant women are particularly vulnerable to gender-based violence. Some husbands become more violent during the wife's pregnancy, even kicking or hitting their wives in the belly. These women run twice the risk of miscarriage and four times the risk of having a low-birth weight baby.

*Rape:* One of the most serious consequences of rape is unwanted pregnancy. Tragically, these women find little support for their condition and face limited options for dealing with the problem in ways that preserve their dignity and provide them with the necessary medical care. They also face exposure to infection from sexually transmitted diseases including HIV/AIDS.

## Looking at Alternate Systems to Treat Common Mental Disorders

The National Mental Health Programme which has three components—Treatment, Rehabilitation and Prevention of illness and Promotion of positive mental health.

### *Treatment*

The treatment programme has been planned keeping the primary health care approach as the sheet anchor. At the same time, it consists of creation of an appropriate referral system at various levels. It is proposed that the specialized psychiatric services should be made available at the district level. The district level health personnel to provide training for the workers at the primary health centre level. The mental hospitals, medical colleges, teaching institutions are linked to the national grid for mental health care particularly in the fields of education and research.

### *Rehabilitation*

This programme is aimed at developing services for the rehabilitation of the chronically disabled due to mental illness as well as mental retardation. This programme envisages links with rehab programmes of other ministries like Social Welfare, and Labour.

*Prevention of Illness and Promotion of Positive Mental Health*

This visualizes counselling services for common mental health problems like alcohol and drug abuse, delinquency and genetically inherited mental illness.

According to Dr. R.S. Murthy the suggestions stated below could be incorporated for the successful implementation of the National Mental Health Programme.

- A decentralized training programme for the existing health personnel on essentials of mental health care at the district level.
- Provision of mental health care in all general health facilities.
- Involvement of all categories of health and welfare personnel in mental health care.
- Provision of essential psychiatric drugs at all health facilities.
- A simple record keeping.
- Mechanisms to monitor the work of primary health care personnel in the provision of mental health care.
- A mental health team at the district level for training of personnel, referral support and supervision of the mental health programme.

Dr. Murthy has emphasised the need for Primary Health Care to be strengthened to face the challenges of treating mental disorders within the community. He further reiterates the concept of Primary Health Care Systems in India as an "approach which aims at integration of all elements of development and welfare to improve the health status of people in the community, it includes preventive, promotive, curative, and rehabilitative measures as well as community developmental activities."

The principles of primary health care are as follows:

- PHC to be shaped around the life pattern of people.

- PHC is an integral part of the health system.
- PHC has to be integrated worth others sectors which are involved in community development and in community welfare like agriculture, rural development, education, labour, communications, social welfare etc.
- Local population is involved in formulation and implementation of PHC.
- Maximum reliance on available community resources is encouraged.
- Integrated approach of preventive, promotive, curative, rehabilitative services for the individuals, family and community.
- Interventions are made at the most peripheral level by suitably trained medical and paramedical workers who are supported by general hospital and consultation hospital personnel.

**Treating Women with Common Disorders in the Community**

The Fourth World Conference on Women, held in Beijing in 1995, specifically endorsed the concept of integrating relevant services for women into primary health care. This implies that the health sector, particularly the reproductive health and family planning sector, needs to more systematically study and respond to the specific health care requirements of victims of gender violence. As the pressure for integrating and decentralising services grows, it will be crucial to create policy reforms that respond to women's specific needs so that appropriate preventive as well as curative programmes are put in place.

Symptomatic treatment will only provide a temporary reprieve if the root causes are not addressed directly. Survivors of gender-based violence do not receive adequate health care until they are critically disabled.

Much of the responsibility for the care of abused women has been delegated by default to small women's organisations, which have neither the resources nor the capacity to fully meet their needs. Yet the health sector is uniquely situated to be an open door to aid for the women who have no other contact with authorities who can help them.

Health care providers can refer women to other resources, such as legal services, safe houses for battered women, and counselling by gender-sensitive NGOs.

**An Alternate Approach to Health Care in Goa**

All Primary Health Care Units should have at least 3 health workers affiliated to it. The Government should look at the finances for the same. Medical personnel, legal personnel and other experts in the field of behavioural and mental health should train the health workers for a period of at least 6 months. The course could comprise of the areas given below. The Directorate of Health Services in collaboration with the resource persons assigned could work out the modules. There should be one person appointed to handle this training in the Directorate of Health Services.

1. Health Education in General.
2. Knowledge of Gynaecological issues.
3. Knowledge of Child Birth, child developmental and other child health related issues.
4. Knowledge of Mental Health issues.
5. Knowledge of different kinds of mental illnesses.
6. Counselling Skills using the problem solving approach.
7. Knowledge of indicators of chronic illness both physical and mental.
8. Knowledge of allied systems available to assist victims of violence.
9. Knowledge of facilities available within the government and the NGO sector, Knowledge of service organisations, care/help groups and help lines available and how to approach the same.
10. Knowledge of resource mapping both in terms of human and services available within the community assigned to the health worker.
11. Knowledge of the use of health advocacy and creative means to spread community awareness of health related issues and its relationship to social issues like alcoholism, family violence, promiscuity etc.

Informative materials and inputs and a resource directory should be a part of the package given to the health workers. From Nos. 4 to 11, if well addressed and trained, the treatment of common mental disorders specifically for women within the community will go a long way.

**Role of a Health Worker**

*Forming a Network of Barefoot Counsellors* : Almost all villages or every second village has a health sub-centre. The health workers then use the sub-centres as a base to meet with barefoot counsellors, agony aunts in the village, old *dais* and nurses or any community people interested in holistic health and forms a health care group in every village.

The health worker is then a facilitator to these groups and s/he in turn learns from them. The group is her/his grass root informant and the community's crises intervention resource person. There is a synergy between these groups and the health worker. These groups have a main agenda every four months, but also attend to other community health issues, for example, alcoholism, the group with the health worker organises talks, films, discussions, street plays etc. on alcoholism but they do not ignore a victim of family violence and will assist her to seek psychological help and social support. Themes sustain the group and the issue is dealt with in depth.

The health workers of each centre are allotted a number of sub-centres under their jurisdiction, which they have to work within with the help of community resource people. They meet formally once a month to take stock of the work done.

*Planning Health Related Activities*

The work should be streamlined into activities such as:

- Crises Intervention;
- Advocacy on Health Related issues and other issues that impact health, through theatre, talks or any medium; the target population need to be school children, teenagers

and adults from the community. Children and teenagers should not be left out.

- *Referrals:* The cases undertaken that needed referrals to allied systems or specialised health care.
- Monitoring of all cases undertaken.
- Record keeping of the activities undertaken and the follow up.
- Conducting workshops on other issues like legal aid, financial schemes, self-employment, which impact the psychological health.

The health worker needs to understand that health is a multi factorial phenomenon and look beyond the symptoms of the target population. S/he needs to involve the whole family and look for permanent solutions to their problems, which will impact the health of the individual who is ill, the family and the community at large.

The health workers can do a lot to improve the quality of life of survivors of family violence, if s/he understands that health is a multi factorial phenomenon and needs the assistance of the police, organisations, employment schemes for destitute women, shelter homes to really work towards improving the health of survivors of violence.

Compassion and zest for bringing about a healthy change in the community should be the attitude of the health worker.

**Extending the Present RCH Programme—Some Suggestions**

Much has been said about the RCH programme to be implemented by July 2003 in an effective and major way within the communities. Maybe one can look at some of the suggestions.

- Innovative approaches to care like looking at alternate systems, *dais,* herbal medicines which have no side effects, meditation, use of yoga etc.
- Development of training in parenting skills to parents of children and adolescents with the assistance of appropriate resource people from NGOs and other service organisations.

- To emphasise on behavioural and psychological health of children along with physical health and incorporate experts in this field to come to PHCs on bimonthly visits so that parents can consult and get assistance.
- Crisis intervention with regard to the health of both women and children.
- Support to HIV/AIDS affected women and post-natal monitoring; screening and prevention of female cancers.
- Counselling facilty with the assistance of experts, for teenagers about responsible sexual behaviour; Health workers also if trained well can assist in this area.
- Counselling about domestic violence and gender equality with the assistance of representatives of NGO'S and counsellors working in this area.
- Fifteen to twenty yearly workshops focus on topics of health, psychology, and legal and social issues for the community.

If RCH programme is to be successful it must incorporate community participation.

### Addressing Gender Violence and Health Care at the Policy Level

Given women's reluctance to report the abuse they are suffering, it is up to health care givers, particularly those in reproductive health services such as antenatal clinics, maternity services, and family planning clinics, to be keenly alert to the possibility that their clients have been abused.

An effective health-care sector response to domestic violence might include the following:

- Forming inter-sectoral working groups to share information and coordinate efforts, made up of health professionals within the community or those from public hospitals (depends on case by case basis) and representatives from local women's organisations, barefoot counsellors, the police and legal aid cells that provide services to victims of violence;

- Training hospital staff in counselling, examining victims, and collecting legal evidence for prosecution;
- Incorporating gender-based violence as a topic in public-health-training curricula for care providers; and
- Developing referral networks and resource materials.

## Community Support for Changes in Better Health

*Efforts of NGOs and Local Organisations:* In Goa there are very few NGOs really looking into the health needs of the people leave alone emphasising on the health of women. It would be effective if organisations and NGOs could see a relation between their work and join hands with the government to address health related issues as a part of their agenda.

*Involving Young People:* A special effort should focus on adolescents. They will be adults and we would like that they grow to be healthy adults. In the area of family adolescents need to develop communication and negotiation skills that will enable them to have intimate relations reflecting these values, particularly in their reproductive and sexual life.

Much of what they see only serves to reinforce gender violence as an acceptable part of their lives. Adolescent boys must be taught that violence against women or girls is not part of their "birthright". Adolescent girls need to be taught about the nature of gender violence—particularly the socialisation process that leads girls to accept this violence as part of being female. They need to be helped to develop self-confidence, self-esteem, and awareness of their reproductive rights. Population/family life education and sex education programmes need to focus on these concerns. Peers and peer counsellors are an important means of reaching out to youth.

*Involving Men:* A large part of the social acceptance of gender-based violence comes from men who essentially see abuse as a male "prerogative". Therefore, changing the mindset of male partners is an important part of the equation for achieving harmony and mutual respect in gender relations. In the Nirmaan Programme we made efforts and although one did not get 100 per cent success it was a beginning.

*Court Counsellors:* A big chunk of our Goan population can be seen making the rounds in courts struggling to get justice. The stress both financially and emotionally costs the public a lot in terms of their health. At least in the area of family problems and family related issues like separation, maintenance, custody of children which are emotionally much more trying than property issues, may be court counsellors will help. Advocate Norma Alvares has mooted this idea and we hope it will see the light of day.

In conclusion, the list of activities to be undertaken to enhance the better health and harmony of the population is unending. It is a myth that Goans are healthy, thanks to the fish and fenny, one is not sure which helps or hinders health but one is sure that common mental disorders specially of women if handled effectively at the community level will impact the same community.

## REFERENCES

Issac, M., Chandrashekhar, C.R. and Murthy, R.S. (1994): *Mental Health Care By Primary Care Doctors,* Bangalore: NIMHANS.

Murthy, R.S.: 'Community Mental Health': 150-176 in Murthy.R.S, *Mental Health in India, 1950-2000, Essays in Honour of Professors N.N.Wig,* Peoples Action for Mental Health (PAMH), Bangalore.

Murthy, R.S.: *Mental Health in India, 1950-2000, Essays in Honour of Professors N.N.Wig,* Peoples Action for Mental Health (PAMH), Bangalore.

UNFPA (1998): Violence Against Girls and Women: A Public Health Priority – Programme Advisory Note, Number 6: Reproductive Health Effects of Gender-Based Violence: Policy and Programme Implications.

# SEX, SEXUALITY AND REPRODUCTIVE HEALTH

# 8

# IMPACT OF TRAFFICKING AND PROSTITUTION ON WOMEN'S HEALTH

## A Case Study of Goa's Baina Beach Red-Light Area

*Arz*

Social and cultural factors including unequal power relations between men and women play primary roles in promoting, protecting or impeding health. Women's health is particularly vulnerable. The social dynamics in a red-light area therefore impacts negatively on the women involved in prostitution and also those merely residing in close proximity to the area. Here women's health status revolves around the dynamics of organised trafficking. This involves the process of submission of women to the norms of the red-light area, exploitative and abusive relationships in the red-light area, violence, extremely unhygienic living conditions, lack of basic sanitation facilities, neglect and stigmatisation, lack of and poor quality of health services, etc. However, it is often the group of women who are residing in a red-light area but not involved in prostitution that go unnoticed and unattended to as much social work and health interventions have focused their attention on women in prostitution.

This paper discusses the vulnerabilities of these two groups of women in the context of Baina Beach red-light area in the state of Goa. It outlines some factors affecting women's health and well-being, and the availability, quality and access to health services. The paper puts forth some recommendations for intervention. Some cases are presented to illustrate the field reality.

## Baina Beach Red-Light Area: The Context for Health Vulnerabilities of the Women

The population of Baina Beach community is approximately 6,000 persons, mostly of ethnic origin of the states of Andhra Pradesh, Karnataka and Uttar Pradesh. Although part of the community is a mobile population, a sizeable portion comprises of persons who are residents of Goa since a period of over three-four decades.

The women of this community are, for the purposes of this paper, sub-divided into women in prostitution and women not in prostitution.

### *Women in Prostitution*

Women in prostitution, include those who are victims/ survivors of prostitution-related trafficking at the Baina Beach red-light area. These women have been trafficked to Goa (either through deceit, physical force or have come due to socio-economic compulsions), a large number of them as minors. Many of them have histories of sexual exploitation, have disadvantaged parental situations, difficult marital circumstances, face societal and gender inequalities, are escaping abusive social or religious customs, or hail from regions affected by natural calamities, ill-effects of globalisation and migration.

A woman, trafficked into prostitution, through any means, undergoes a process of coping with prostitution throughout her life cycle within it. During this, she experiences varying degrees of trauma and adopts different coping mechanisms, all of which leave a deep psychological impact on her. Women, whether they have arrived in the red-light area knowingly or otherwise, are often unable to acknowledge the reality of the situation of being prostituted when faced with it. The non-acceptance creates situations where there is a dichotomy between the compulsion to accept reality and a desire to escape, which manifests itself through various disorders like acute depression, schizophrenia and stress related syndromes. Unable to find any means of escape from the situation physically or psychologically, attempts such as suicide are often perceived as the only way out for them. Many women in prostitution have wrists scarred with razor cuts. Lack of focus on mental health of prostituted women as well as a lack of services directed towards such issues have only worsened the situation.

Baina Beach red-light area for many women in prostitution is an alien surrounding where the culture, language, geography of the area are unfamiliar to them. This thus compels them to be dependent on their perpetrators, leading to extreme exploitation.

Brothel-keepers exploit women in prostitution with a view to earn maximum profits and to retain them in debt bondage and prostitution. The women in prostitution who are under a brothel-keeper are usually driven to prostitute without respite and under the directions of the brothel-keeper. This results in various forms of exploitation and risky sexual practices. Besides, the earnings of the girls are deliberately miscalculated by brothel-keepers to reflect large unpaid amounts. The girls are not allowed to shift brothels and live with fear and threats of arrest by the police. Physically too their movement is kept highly restricted. The alien surroundings, unknown language, and dependence on escorts to move around hinder their access to various services including health-care.

Women in prostitution face extreme violence. A woman in prostitution is not treated as an individual with rights but as an object for commercial sex. Therefore, violence towards her is not treated as a crime. Since most prostituted women are in debt-bondage, it also becomes difficult for them to register their protest when any act of physical and sexual violence like rape or assault takes place.

The prostituted women also face harassment at the hands of their 'parasitical' male-keeps (or 'mards' as they are more popularly known) who use these women simply as a source of economic and physical sustenance. The initial need to have male-keeps is motivated by peer pressure and the desire for emotional and physical security, as well as to gain a sense of self-worth, but soon the relationship becomes exploitative in nature. The male-keep indulges in multiple sexual relationships, addictions, and excessive demands on the woman to prostitute at the same time restrictions on her interactions with customers. This further develops into emotional blackmail, battering, excessive sexual demands, and threats of harm or arrest when the woman wants an exit out of the relationship. Violent behaviour is not treated as an issue of concern and more often than not goes unreported. Also, given the helplessness of their situation, the women are unable to ask for help, endangering their emotional, physical and sexual health in the process. Another aspect of the male-keep relationship is the non-use of condoms in sexual interactions with the male keep. Women do not have protected sex with male keeps as it is treated as a marital relationship, however male-keeps frequently change partners, making the women very vulnerable to HIV infections.

The red-light area has a sub-culture of its own. These sub-cultural norms have to be endured by the woman in prostitution such as forced sexual interactions with women in prostitution, physical abuse by perpetrators, consumption of alcohol or performance of perverse sexual acts as demanded by the customer, the right of the male-keep to have multiple partnerships. This makes her susceptible to situations of health vulnerabilities ranging from mental trauma, sexually transmitted diseases and HIV.

The physical act of prostitution itself takes a toll on her physical as well as mental health. The act of indulging in multiple sexual activity, often unprotected sexual activity and early initiation into it to earn one's living (since most women are introduced to the profession when they are still minors), carries with it a burden of various illnesses, some serious and life-threatening. Some of the diseases that are treated more as occupational hazards are STD's like gonorrhoea, syphilis, genital warts, and genital herpes. Repeated and continuous sexual intercourse over a period of time also exposes these women to complications of pelvic inflammatory diseases that in turn carry greater risks of cervical cancer. Multiple abortions, which start from early adolescence further impede their reproductive health.

Added to all this is the lack of awareness of law, lack of support from local population, intimidation by police and anti-social elements which increases their situation of helplessness.

The resultant stress leads to addictive habits, aggressive and self-destructive behaviour such as frequent suicide attempts, involvement in abusive relationships, and in the long-term development into abusers or perpetrators themselves.

The woman in prostitution over a period of time is left to fight for her own survival. She is left without her fair share of earnings, gets involved in various abusive relationships, is indebted for large amounts of money, borrows to fulfill the needs of her dependants, is intimidated by members of the prostitution market, is confronted constantly with all forms of stigmatisation, finds herself trapped perpetually in prostitution, sees no alternatives to change her situation and adapts various unproductive means to cope with her stress and trauma. The environment of the red-light area which is characterised by extreme violence, aggression, abuse and addictions is the source for her learning of coping mechanisms ranging from physical abuse, self-destruction to engagement in addiction. There is an overall resignation to one's life-situation, lack of hope in change and hence lack of will to access or accept services towards the same.

### *Women not in Prostitution*

Women not in prostitution are those who are not associated with the dynamics of the prostitution market but reside in and around the red-light area by way of being born or married there, or who have migrated to the area for other reasons. Although not directly involved in the prostitution market, they are also psychologically, physically and socially affected by mere proximity to the red light area. These women find it stressful to adjust to the surroundings and cope with the norms of the red-light area.

The spouses of these women are often involved in extra-marital affairs or continue pre-marital relationships mostly with prostituted women. The engagement in sexual interaction with prostituted women habituates the husband to certain forms of sexual behaviour and builds certain images of sexual interaction that are imposed upon the spouse not in prostitution. Many a times women find themselves unable to cope with the demands of their husbands. Inability or refusal to yield to such requirements results in women being victims of aggression, physical and sexual assault. The husband's extra-marital relationships also lead to a spread in infections from the husband to the wife, such as HIV, STD's and T.B.

The extra-marital relationships of their husbands invariably leads to financial instability in the family. Many a times, it becomes nearly impossible to run the household and the woman is forced to look for some means to earn a living and support her children. There are also instances where her earnings become a support for her husband's addictions. The nature of work that the woman generally finds is as a helper in the red-light area or as a rag-picker, both of which make the woman exposed to further violence and abuse.

A basic feature of the living conditions, common to both groups of women, is the near total absence of even the most basic facilities like water, sanitation and hygiene. Lack of proper waste disposal and drainage system, frequent water-logging, lack of ventilation in the rooms only make the place a breeding ground for malaria, typhoid and other water-borne diseases. The sanitary concerns of women are heightened in view of the compulsion to use the open beach area as a toilet as the only public toilet servicing the entire community is fee-based and unaffordable by the entire family. The compulsion for women to access an open area forces them to restrict attendance to their sanitary needs to specific times such as early morning or in the darkness of the evening when there are fewer men around. The continued use of the same area predisposes them to infections.

Lastly, the overall 'unempowered' status of the woman at Baina Beach itself becomes an impediment to health and well being. The fact that the woman is not sufficiently empowered, and is always under the control of perpetrators denies her access to medical care or completion of treatment of any illness she suffers from despite the awareness of the availability of services.

## Community Response to Health Issues of Women

Health concerns of women are not the community's priority at Baina Beach. Treatment and care, especially in the case of women, are postponed till they become necessary for survival. Responsible causes range from insensitivity to women's issues, control of women in prostitution by perpetrators, financial reasons, lack of family or community support in times of health crisis, health not perceived as a basic need for all round growth and development.

Another important feature of the poor health conditions in Baina is women's unwillingness to access health care services outside Baina for fear of stigmatisation. Due to the stigmatisation faced in the local public health services, families often end up not reporting illnesses since accessing private health care becomes quite costly. This has been seen to happen on four levels: (*a*) geographical background—stigmatisation merely because of their belonging to Baina red-light area; (*b*) occupation—for practising prostitution; (*c*) disease—the assumption that anyone from that area is HIV positive; and (*d*) ethnicity—for being migrants from Uttar Pradesh, Karnataka, etc. Such stigmatisation has had obvious detrimental effects on access of health-care services in Baina.

Negative experiences with the health services has further worsened the situation in the community. The community now has its own share of preconceived notions and myths about the working of the health system, that is large hospitals like the Goa Medical College. Continued maltreatment of the people of Baina Beach only results in the perpetuation of these myths.

### *Health Services*

For the women at Baina Beach, health services are available through Government, private and voluntary organisations.

The existence of government health services with adequate infrastructure and facilities within the red-light area is negligible. As already mentioned, other health services do not always provide complete and sustainable systems of health care for women in the Baina Beach community.

Due to the activities of prostitution carried on here, the migrant status of its residents, their economic and social situation, the women of Baina Beach, irrespective of their occupation or location of residence, are treated with disgust, disdain and ostracism from persons residing outside the area. In the context of health services, they face a discriminatory attitude from government health officials. On the other hand, private health services close to the red-light area flourish as perpetrators are willing to pay high rates for medical care. This makes access of these services difficult for women not in prostitution and exploitative for women in prostitution in terms of extended debt-bondage as they have to repay the medical bills in double to the perpetrators. This plays a very strong role in the deprivation of the health facilities for the women of this community.

Further, it is difficult to find residential and outreach services in areas of de-addiction, mental health care, and shelter for prostituted women who are victims of violence, HIV positive women etc. Special services like pre and post-test HIV counselling services are infrequently provided to women and families affected with HIV. Being afflicted with the HIV virus is dreaded not only because of it's incurable nature, but also because of the prohibitive social and economic costs that go along with it, in terms of ostracism and the high costs of medication, which are often beyond the reach of the affected group. In Baina Beach, there are no long-term comprehensive and sustainable health services available. There is a lack of dissemination of information for instance on reproductive health rights for mothers, or the spread of TB and STD's. There is also a lack of willingness to do case follow-ups in a red-light area as part of outreach services of the government health system.

The stigmatisation of women of Baina Beach by health practitioners has forced women to use unsafe and unscientific methods for alleviating health problems. For example they often practice risky abortion methods, which further endangers the health of the women.

Health services provided by voluntary organisations include free distribution and social marketing of condoms, awareness regarding HIV/AIDS and more recently services for general illnesses as well. Services such as HIV testing, diagnosis, limited treatment and referrals are also provided.

Services provided by the voluntary sector are largely curative. This implies that ultimately the community at a later stage of any illness have to go to government services for medical attention.

**Case No. 1 : Prostitution a Cause of Mental Ill-Health**

Laxmi was in her early twenties, a destitute with two children. Her entry into the red-light area had primarily been to support her children. She fell prey to mental health problems primarily as a consequence of her inability to cope with the demands of prostitution. She was never comfortable with the idea of selling herself for sex with different men, whom she would not otherwise choose to have relationships with. This caused her immense mental disturbance. Yet Laxmi could not find alternatives to escape. This resulted in a loss of self-esteem. The gap between the demands of her real self and the demands of the prostitution market kept widening, a gap that she could not deal with in her day-to-day life.

What began as a coping mechanism grew into an addiction. Her attempt to cope with her situation was to addict herself to alcohol. She frequently tried to run away from her brothel and the red-light area. At times when she did this, she would lose all sense of herself. She would return to her past life and reiterate the experiences of her life that brought back positive memories, which provided her a sense of comfort and re-established her self-esteem for a brief period of time. As soon as her mind returned to the present, she would consume more alcohol to blank out her experiences.

She was then unable to carry out her daily functions and her behaviour affected others around her as she would often have fights with other women, her male-keep and her brothel-keeper. She was unable to take care of her children's basic needs. In extreme disturbing moments Laxmi would strip off her clothes in public places and at other times attempt to commit suicide by walking into the sea. As her mental disturbance worsened, she became a recluse, had conversations with herself was not able to look after her own personal needs.

With the help of Arz, the community and the police, Laxmi was admitted to the Government Institute for Psychiatric and Human Behaviour (IPHB) at Altinho, Panjim. There, Laxmi felt she was stigmatised by the para-medical staff for being 'a woman from Baina', a prostituted woman. It was always assumed that she was a HIV patient and that was what was repeatedly told to her. She agonized that she was not treated with basic human dignity or as an equal. She had been detained in a ward that housed patients suffering from a range of mental health problems. Laxmi could not accept her classification in the category of other extreme mental health patients.

This caused Laxmi to repel all attempts of counselling made by the doctors. She was finally released from the Institution with advice for follow up. Laxmi had benefited from the admission to a limited extent. Laxmi rejected any attempts of follow up at IPHB as she did not want to re-visit her negative experiences at the Institute. There were no outreach facilities available at Baina Beach to which Laxmi could be referred. When Laxmi returned to the red-light she developed the same symptoms of earlier mental disturbance. In her last attempt to run away from the red-light area, she returned to her village, where she died. Laxmi had died at a very young age, leaving her two children orphaned.

### Case No. 2 : Even Women Who are not in Prostitution are Stigmatized

Rita is 25-year-old has been residing at Baina Beach since her childhood. Her husband who is an alcoholic, engaged in multiple sexual relationships in the red-light area, often physically assaults her. Rita sells vegetables herself to supplement her family income.

Rita has had 4 children, aged 8, 5, 3 and 1 year respectively, in 9 years of marriage. Rita delivered all her children born at home. No Trained Birth Attendants (TBAs) have attended on her. She has not been able to afford private health care. Although she visited the local government hospital for her monthly check-ups in her last pregnancy, she finally had her delivery at home. During her visits to the local hospital, she found herself being stigmatised because of her migrant status, her poor economic condition, as well as her residence at Baina Beach. She was never even informed by the government health functionaries of the availability of contraception.

### Case No. 3 : Interventions Can Help

Sarita was prostituted in her early thirties and returned to the red-light area after her five year marriage broke up. She was then suffering from Tuberculosis. Although she returned to the red-light area, Sarita did not want to rejoin prostitution and approached Arz for employment. She was however unable to work due to her health problem. Sarita lost the employment opportunity. She was admitted to the Government T.B. Hospital in Panaji where she was also diagnosed to be HIV positive. She underwent hospitalisation and was discharged with requirement for long-term treatment for T.B.

On her return to the red-light area, she began consumption of alcohol, did not take regular medication, was incapable of engaging in any other gainful employment for her support and had to engage in prostitution for survival.

Continuity in medical treatment was also affected by the absence of the facility to administer T.B. medications at the closest Government Hospital and the compulsion to collect the same from the T.B. Hospital at Panaji. Sarita would find it difficult to be regular for her medical replenishments due to factors such as distance, inability to sponsor her travel, her continued alcohol intake, her failing health as well as sometimes her inability to read the medical card. There were no follow-ups or outreach facilities of the Government medical system close to Baina Beach. In instances of travel being sponsored by Arz, Sarita was not inclined to travel the long distance for follow up. There was a lack of inclination to continue treatment.

Sarita became involved in a relationship with a male-keep in the area. She felt she had to continue prostitution to support herself and her male-keep. The controlling influence of the male-keep was very strong. He exercised all means to keep Sarita in the red-light area, even if it meant her deteriorating health, as he depended on her income. He even interfered with her medical treatment at hospital and influenced Sarita to discontinue her hospitalization.

Sarita's health gradually declined. She refused to continue the treatment. Her continued prostitution in the face of HIV infection also contributed to her further deteriorated health status.

Arz attempted to seek facilities for her shelter away from the red-light area. However, on the one hand there was resistance from Sarita due to her dependence on the male-keep, resistance from the male-keep who controlled her and pretended to be her genuine caretaker and on the other hand the absolute absence of any shelter in the state that was open to admitting a prostituted woman who is an HIV patient.

In time, the male-keep was arrested for previous criminal record. His separation from Sarita allowed Arz to intervene to empower Sarita and make her understand the need to take care of her health needs. Sarita is now residing in a residential facility away from the red-light area. She is continuing her T.B. treatment. Arz does continued follow up.

## Some Factors Affecting Women's Health Status in Baina, Red-Light Area

### *Trafficking*

The occurrence of trafficking for an individual who is a victim has implications for the health of the individual. The process of being commodified impacts on the psychology of the victim. This is worse in the case of women who have been trafficked through deceit.

*Exploitation and Bondage*

The situation of a woman in prostitution characterised by exploitation and bondage predisposes her to health vulnerabilities. By virtue of her being in the control of her perpetrators, decisions regarding her health needs as well as access to health services are made by her exploiters. Health services delivered to her are used as a tool for further exploitation and debt-bondage.

*Prostitution Market*

The process of 'socialisation' that a woman in prostitution undergoes in order to adapt to the situation in the market has effects on her health. The nature of her ability to adapt to the idea of being on sale for sex, soliciting, adapting to changed dressing styles, language and behaviour, etc. largely has direct implications for her health status.

*Frequent Intercourse with Multiple Sex Partners*

Engagement in frequent, multiple sexual intercourse exposes women in prostitution to various illnesses which can take serious and life-threatening turns. Repeated and continuous sexual intercourse over a period of time also exposes these women to complications that carry greater risks of health. Multiple abortions, which start from early adolescence greatly impede their reproductive health.

*Introduction of Women into Prostitution as Minors*

The introduction of women into prostitution as minors carries effects into adulthood. Minors in prostitution do not have skills to cope with the prostitution market and therefore are easily exploited. Resultant psychological, physical and sexual harm caused at an early age, continues to afflict individual women in prostitution right to adulthood. For example, younger girls being more in demand in the flesh-trade, the perpetrator profits more by offering them for engagement in frequent unguarded multiple commercial sexual intercourse resulting in multiple abortions, which start from early adolescence. Dangerous, delayed and multiple abortions carry their effects on the woman's reproductive health into her adult life.

*Occupational Pressures*

By virtue of being in prostitution, certain behaviour enforced upon women in prostitution such as compulsion to perform perverse sex, engage in unprotected sex, engagement in addictive habits such as smoking, consumption of alcohol, serving large number of customers per day, prostitution throughout the month without sufficient breaks, create long-term health risks.

*Violence*

The excessive and frequent violence in the red-light area by brothel-keepers, pimps, amongst prostituted women, customers, male-keeps, police, itself predisposes the woman in prostitution to psychological as well as physical damage.

*Sub-cultural Acceptance*

The red-light area is a sub-culture of its own. Certain behaviour considered acceptable by the sub-cultural community such as susceptibility of the woman in prostitution to sexual infections, the right of the male to have multiple partnerships, forced sexual interactions with women in prostitution, physical abuse by perpetrators, double repayment system, puts a woman into situations of health vulnerabilities.

*Male-keeps*

The necessity for a woman in prostitution to keep a male-keep owing to risks and social situations inherent in the red-light area, predisposes the woman in prostitution to health hazards. The invariable deterioration of the relationship into emotional blackmail, extreme physical abuse, excessive sexual demands, multiple sexual relationships of the male-keep, continued financial dependence of the male-keep and the non-use of condoms in sexual interactions with the male-keep causes direct effects on the health of the woman.

*No Participation in Decision-Making*

The low empowered status of the women directly leading to their inability to make decisions for their well-being, is a significant factor contributing to health risks and deterioration. The woman finds herself unable to take decisions or steps also in terms of other aspects of her life-situation which lends to worsened health status.

*Low Self-Esteem*

Owing to her status of being prostituted, the low self-esteem, disinterest in life, lack of optimism, low or no expectancy of better opportunities directly leads to a lack of interest in improving her health situation.

*Accumulation of Experiences of Mistrust and Dependence of Others*

The life-view of a woman in prostitution due to a series of occurrences of breach of trust, cheating and 'parasitical' dependence of those around her affects her will to improve her health and access to health services.

*Dependence on Exploiters*

Dependence on perpetrators being the most commonly adopted

recourse of a woman in prostitution during crisis leads to further exploitation thus also vulnerability in terms of health.

*Indebtedness*

The large degree of indebtedness that women in prostitution are constantly pressurised by directly affects their will to access health services. Many a times, the possibility of having to repay the brothel-keeper double or inflated bill amounts restricts their will to express health disabilities.

*Substance Abuse*

Easy and cheap availability of addictive substances (alcohol, ghutka, addictive tablets) is another factor that leads already stressed women to substance dependence, which lead them into complications of health and life threatening situations.

*Self Harm Due to Inability to Cope*

The responses of the woman in prostitution during times of crises lead her to further victimisation and health-risk situations. For instance, with excessively stressful situations in the red-light area women have even resorted to slashing of their wrists and forearms in their inability to handle situations.

*Lack of Awareness of Services*

The lack of awareness of prostituted women regarding health facilities is a significant cause for vulnerability to health problems.

*Language*

The lack of knowledge of local languages and the lack of literacy of the women directly affects her accessibility and nature of health service provided to her.

### *Sexual Behaviour Patterns in the Area*

Existent sexual behaviour patterns in the community have a direct detrimental effect on the health of women. Women are prone to extreme health hazards through some sexual behaviour patterns such as the multiple sexual partnership of male-keeps, the continued sexual interaction of married men in the community with prostituted women, the non-usage of condoms by the spouse or male-keep with the woman, the prostituted woman's pattern of condom use affected by her perception of the relationship with her male-keep as a marital relationship.

### *Stigmatisation*

Stigmatisation is an all-encompassing factor affecting the health of the women, both those in and not in prostitution. The extremely stigmatised treatment meted out in hospitals and repeated experiences of stigmatisation affects the accessibility of health services.

### *Non-Availability of Adequate Health Services*

Inherent flaws in the organisation of health services especially government health services such as the lack of outreach, lack of decentralised local outlets of health services, absence of monitoring and follow up mechanisms and the insufficient spread of the health network has that directly affected the health status of women at Baina Beach.

### *Poor Health Service Delivery*

The health status of the women at Baina Beach has a strong direct linkage with poor quality of health service reaching them such as irregularity of medical staff, delays in service provision, long periods of waiting, rude and unconcerned behaviour, insufficient dispense of free medication, inefficient information-provision, discrimination.

*Dependence on Non-Government Health Services*

The dependence of women on non-government health services becomes a factor that hampers their well-being when the nature of service required by the women is not within the capacities of the non-government service and when the women have lost the will to recommence contact with government health services.

*Past Experiences with Health Services*

The accumulation of the community's as well as individual woman's experiences with health service providers shapes her perceptions of the health service and directly affects her future utilisation of that service. In the case of Baina Beach, the experiences largely being negative, the woman's perception of health services is mostly negative and it causes the resistance to access these services even in emergency and crisis situations.

*Physical Environment of the Area*

The physical environment of cramped living quarters, with no facilities for proper ventilation as well as sanitation, no systems of drainage or periodic garbage cleaning systems or even proper community toilet facilities has direct implications for health problems of women.

*Economic Status of Family*

The poor economic status in the context of expensive private health facilities, lack of availability of free medication dispensed by government health services directly affects the health status of women at Baina Beach. Other factors that affect health of women such as location of the free health services, distance to be travelled and the loss of earnings in trying to access these services in view of the status of most women being daily earners.

*Myths and Rigid Perceptions*

The long-term beliefs either in myths or general perceptions of health services directly affects the access of health services and hence probability of improvement in the health situation of women at Baina Beach.

*Gender Discrimination*

The common phenomenon of women by virtue of their gender, facing a less preferred status in the family or community and thus affecting the status of health concerns also affects the women at Baina Beach. Also, the lack of health related attention provided to them as girl-children leaves an impact on their health as an adult.

*Communal Lack of Priority for Health*

Health being an issue of low priority as a whole for the community of Baina Beach directly affects the health of the community, most importantly that of women.

*Impoverishment-Led Lack of Communal Responsibility or Participation*

The lack of community members' participation in ensuring the well-being or helping each other in times of need becomes a factor that affects the health vulnerabilities of individual members, including women. In case of women in prostitution, their status as single unattached members in the community creating situations of having no escorts, accompaniment or caretaker discourages them to take complete or residential treatment such as hospitalisation.

## Recommendations for Action Towards the Prevention of Health Vulnerabilities and Promotion of Holistic Health for Women at Baina Beach

The health status of any person is intricately linked with the life situation of that person. Interventions in the area of health cannot be carried out in isolation without the consideration of the context of the persons for whom interventions are made. Health interventions therefore in a red-light area where trafficking exists, should preferably focus on the issues of exploitation, discrimination, and the disadvantaged socio-economic status which contributes to ill-health. The health related interventions should be carried out in consonance with interventions related to trafficking and exploitation within prostitution. Health is the responsibility of the State, only the State can provide a sustainable means of well-being for its people and Government Health Services should be available to all equally and without discrimination.

- Health should not be treated in isolation from other issues. Key issues like trafficking, dedication of minor girls, exploitation by the systems etc., which serve to keep women in the flesh trade, should also be addressed as part of the intervention process in health. State action should be planned and implemented against traffickers. Existing laws against trafficking should be implemented and enactment of laws such as a State Devadasi Abolishment Act should be done. Special initiatives should be taken towards identification and rescue of minors in the red-light area.
- State action should be taken to remove situations of debt bondage in prostitution and create conditions to enable women to take their own decisions. State systems especially law enforcing systems must be activated to stop exploitation of women in the area. Channels of non-intimidated recourse to law enforcers and access of law by women should be developed to prevent further victimisation and action taken should be victim-friendly.
- All efforts should be made to stop Child Trafficking and Prostitution at Baina Beach.
- Violence against women, in any form, should be treated as a serious health issue, and its effects should be distinctly monitored and addressed through providing free legal services, shelter homes, and counselling to cope with the emotional trauma. Simultaneously, key figures like the

husbands, the brothel-keepers, the customers and the mards must be made a part of such awareness programmes. The local police need to be sensitive to the issue of violence and take victim-oriented approach.

- Violence against any woman, also women in prostitution, detected by any health agency, should be reported to the Police for action.
- Police should be sensitised regarding the health implications of violence, exploitation and trafficking on women.
- Health systems should be made stigmatisation-free at all levels of health staff hierarchy. Attitudinal change in the government personnel through awareness and sensitisation programmes must be carried out. A system of monitoring attitudes and behaviour of health staff must be enforced. Systems for reporting stigmatisation should be developed and action taken against persons indulging in stigmatory practices.
- The health system should be made sensitive to the issue of prostitution and accept these women as victims of an already exploitative situation and not put her through any kind of labelling.
- State Health department should devise procedures of detection and action against any exploitation of women (such as excessive charges, conduct of unnecessary medical tests, collusion with perpetrators, etc.) caused by non-government or private medical practitioners. A system of redressal should be established for women facing exploitation by health service providers.
- The system of health service delivery of the STD clinic should be re-organised and upgraded to the status of a Primary Health Centre. The services of the clinic should not be restricted to treatment of STD's and HIV/AIDS but should be extended to provide medical help for all types of illnesses and to all women of the community. The clinic should be enabled to provide 24 hours service. The clinic should be equipped with better infrastructure, equipment and materials such as communication systems,

better laboratory, ambulance or system of sharing ambulance with Chicalim Government Hospital, updated stock of medication and have minimal bed facilities.

- The purview of service-delivery of the local STD clinic should be widened to include mental health services, services for alcoholism, dispense of TB medication, community outreach for follow up, direct referrals to medical services of specialised nature such as TB Hospitals. Doctors and para-medical staff should be available on duty during stipulated working hours.
- Health service provision should be holistic and encompass all areas of self-development. Health centres must include services of counselling, information-provision, recreation, linkages with other government services such as I.C.D.S., provision of alternate health services such as yoga, etc. towards promotion of all-round mental and physical health of women.
- A Special Outpost of Mental Health must be established at Baina Beach with a comprehensive mental health programme for women including local provision of counselling and psychiatric services to the women at Baina Beach as well as monitoring and follow up services.
- Communication with patients at the Baina Government Health Clinic, not conversant in local languages, must be ensured in their native language *i.e.* Kannada and Telugu and not through perpetrators as medium of translation.
- Awareness provision must be more comprehensive and carried out on a regular basis. Awareness should include the preventive aspect of different health care (besides STDs and HIV), along with awareness on curative information *i.e.* spreading awareness and disseminating information on the spread of diseases as well as treatment available.
- Awareness should include increased effort to cover and address the key power structures through the programmes, like brothel-keepers, pimps, mards, husbands of community women since they play an important role in deciding a woman's well-being. Awareness programmes should also include these groups.

- Health service provision must include focus on other common illnesses of the community such as TB, reproductive health, pediatric health care, general health problems and alleviation of direct causal factors.
- Immediate needs of the women of Baina Beach in terms of improvement of civic amenities at Baina Beach in terms of more number of public toilets, facilities for drinking water, efficient waste disposal system should be carried out.
- Reproductive health services should receive increased attention. Women should be given enough information to be able to make informed choices about the use of family planning methods, and key family members should be targeted to generate awareness. Reproductive health runs the whole gamut of safe pregnancy, pre-and post-natal care, ration for pregnant and lactating mothers, so the focus should shift from its incessant glare on family planning and instead should focus on strengthening the basic government infrastructures to ensure a healthy mother and a healthy baby. Greater awareness of measures of contraception should be carried out. Awareness should not be limited only to condom-use but should cover the range of contraceptive methods thus giving the opportunity of informed choices to women.
- A comprehensive de-addiction programme should be implemented in the red-light area for patients of alcoholism. Facilities such as substance-abuse counselling and group sessions must be provided in the red-light area. Post-detoxification residential facilities for women must be made available in the State.
- The work on HIV/AIDS interventions must include simultaneous work on rights interventions in terms of awareness of the woman's rights, referrals in situations of rights violations, support to women for rights assertion.
- The focus of HIV/AIDS interventions should be intensified on groups primarily responsible for the spread of the virus in the red-light area such as male-keeps, customers, brothel-keepers.

- At no cost, should the services of perpetrators be entailed in the provision or implementation of health services, whether creation of awareness, follow up, referrals, distribution of condoms, mobilisation for voluntary blood testing, etc.
- Voluntary Health Interventions should emphasise on mobilization of community participation and building community responsibility related to community health. Interventions that could cause dependence on voluntary service that do not include long-term treatment and care should be avoided. The emphasis on health focused organisations in the community should be to enable, strengthen and create sustainable systems of access of Government services. NGOs should participate in strengthening Government health services.
- Framing of health policies must include special focus on groups such as women in and around red-light areas and their specific health disabilities in the context of the particular disadvantages of being a woman in a developing country and its role in the restriction of access to basic health care.
- Gender blind policies should be refocused on providing gender sensitive health care services that directly address the particular health needs of women.

# 9

# GENDER-LINKED VULNERABILITIES IN THE HIV/AIDS CONTEXT

*Mariette Correa*

In the initial stages of the AIDS pandemic, it was believed that homosexuals and intravenous drug users were the groups at greatest risk of contracting HIV. Gradually, the rates of heterosexual transmission increased. While men still account for the majority of those infected by HIV, the proportion of women being infected over the years is steadily increasing.

By the end of 2001 an estimated 40 million people (of whom 17.6 million were women and 2.7 million were children under 15) had been infected with HIV globally. According to WHO estimates approximately 14,000 new infections occur each day. It is also said that as a direct outcome of mother-to-child transmission, infant and child deaths will increase by as much as 30 per cent by the year 2010.

The fact that HIV/AIDS poses a greater threat to women and girls is now undisputed. In 1997, women represented 41 per cent of adults infected with HIV; by 2000 this figure had reached 47 per cent. Therefore, of the 36.1 million people estimated to be living with HIV/AIDS across the world, 16.4 million are women, 18.3 million are men and 1.4 million are children.

Given the increased susceptibility of HIV+ women to illnesses, their lack of access to care and support, it is not surprising to note that out of the 21.8 million people estimated to have died of AIDS by 2000, the number of women is more than men. (9 million women, 8.5 million men, 4.3 million children).

**The Impact of HIV/AIDS on the World's women, men, and children***

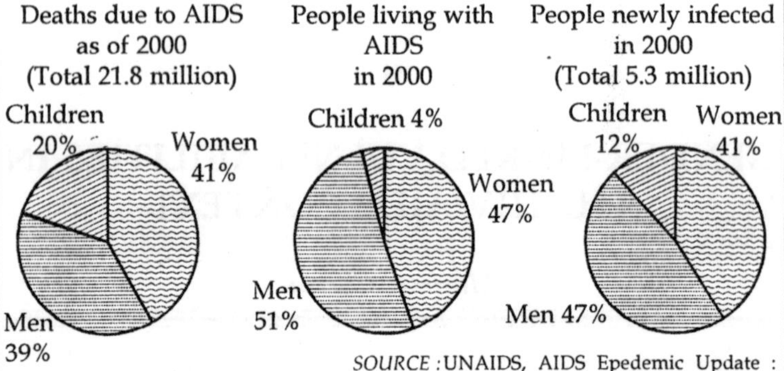


* aged 15 and younger

*SOURCE* : UNAIDS, AIDS Epedemic Update : December 2000, Geneva UNAIDS 2000

There is enough data to show that developing countries are far more vulnerable, and marginalised groups within these still more so. Within the developing countries, India accounts for an estimated 3.97 million of all the people infected with HIV, the southern states being particularly hard hit. At the end of 2001, India's adult HIV prevalence rate was just under 1 per cent. Goa, which lies on the south-west coast of India, is surrounded by high prevalent states. While the percentage of those infected in Goa still does not seem high, *i.e.* less than 1 per cent of the total population, the actual numbers of HIV+ cases in the State are alarming considering the small population of Goa. Moreover, the rate of infection seems to keep increasing though recent trends show that the rate of increase has slowed down. While it is still too premature to gauge the statistical significance of this data, there is no real room for complacency.

Women in developing countries are much more at risk and affected by the pandemic. The situation in Goa is reflective of the global trend, where the proportion of women infected is increasing over the years. Where the sex ratio is concerned, clear data is available only from the 90's where it can be seen that almost 75 per cent of those infected were men. In 1997, where for every woman infected there were three infected men, in 2001 women account for one out of every three people infected.

> **UNAIDS 2001, Gender and AIDS, Almanac, Fact Sheet**
>
> Last year 1.3 million women died of AIDS. Over 16.4 million women today are living with HIV/AIDS.
>
> In Sub-Saharan Africa, teenage girls are 5 times more likely to be infected than boys, since girls are mostly infected not by boys their own age, but by older men.
>
> In surveys in 17 countries, over half of the girls could not name a method of protection against HIV transmission.
>
> 55 per cent of all HIV positive adults in Sub-Saharan Africa are women.
>
> In the last three years, the percentage of people infected with HIV that are women has risen from 41 to 47 per cent.
>
> A UNIFEM study in Senegal showed that the combination of availability, training in the use of female condoms and training in negotiating skills resulted in 80 per cent of the women being able to protect themselves from unsafe sex.
>
> In India, a UNIFEM survey revealed that many women experienced neglect by the medical staff who refused to touch them, or give them injections. Some said they were tested without consent and in many cases, their sero status was shared with their family members also without their consent.

### Reasons for Women' Vulnerability

There are several reasons for women's increasing vulnerability including biological, socio-cultural, political and socio-economic factors.

### Biological

Physiologically, women have a greater chance of contracting

the virus from a man than *vice-versa.* This is due to a larger exposure of mucous membrane within a woman's genital area as well as the high concentration of HIV in the semen as compared to vaginal fluids. In cultures where men prefer 'dry sex', which inhibits women's secretions during sexual intercourse, the chances of trauma of the vaginal canal and tearing are high. Young girls who are sexually exploited are at even greater risk as their genital tracts are still not developed; the cervix is immature and the vaginal walls are thin. Rape and violent sex also increase the efficiency of HIV transmission. Anal intercourse, though rarely discussed is a common sexual practice during menstruation and as contraception. The lack of strong condoms for anal intercourse and the greater chances of rupture of mucous membrane during anal intercourse further increase the risk to women.

STDs and RTIs in women often go undetected, increasing women's risk to HIV. There are many other health problems faced by women in developing countries which predispose them to blood transfusions including chronic anaemia, complicated pregnancies and unsafe abortions. HIV positive women who become pregnant may pass on the virus to their babies before, during or after delivery.

**Socio-cultural**

Women's vulnerabilities are enhanced by the inequalities and discrimination to which they are subjected in patriarchal societies. This includes their lack of access to information, education and health services, and their inability to negotiate safer sexual practices even within marriage.

Research has shown that the lack of knowledge and misconceptions about AIDS is much higher among women than men. In addition, women and especially young girls have very little knowledge about their own bodies. This, together with a low self-esteem about sexuality so common among girls and perpetuated in male-dominated structures, means that women are unable to talk about leave alone negotiate safe sex.

Cultural and traditional values are one of the main barriers to frank and open discussion on HIV/AIDS especially in some parts of the world. With women and young girls this is even more so. As a result most women are denied information and services that can assist them in checking the spread of the disease.

The gender inequalities in what is considered culturally acceptable further reduce the ability of women to discuss their sexuality. For instance, it would be practically a violation of cultural norms for women in many cultures to insist on condom use. Thus, while the female condom and microbicides are being developed in order to enable women to have choices, these technical solutions ignore the fact that women are still powerless to negotiate for safe sex due to their low status.

Women with STDs are often scared or ashamed to seek treatment due to risk of social and familial condemnation. This is compounded by the low importance women give their own health.

Women with HIV/AIDS face many problems different from men, many of which are related to the way society views these women. Due to both ignorance about the modes of transmission and moral connotations attached to HIV, women are discriminated against far more than men. While for men sexual 'adventures' are considered acceptable both before and after marriage, for women they are not. The discrimination women face range from social isolation to verbal and physical abuse to gross violation of fundamental rights.

Many women who become infected with HIV are monogamous and have no perceived risks; they are unaware of the fact that they have contracted the virus till their partners get AIDS, after the death of their partners or if they have an HIV related illness.

Cultural practices that increase the vulnerability of girls ranging from early marriage to female genital mutilation are still practiced in some parts of the world.

Another serious problem which is still not given adequate attention is the problem of drug abuse. It is gradually being accepted that women particularly in developing countries face greater problems from drug misuse than men do. This is exemplified in a study done in India by the United Nations International Drug Control Programme and India's Ministry of Social Justice and Empowerment, which shows that misuse of drugs has a serious impact on women as mothers, wives, and sisters of misusers. "Such an impact becomes even more serious in a developing country like India where women are already disadvantaged," says the report. Women are subjected to domestic violence often in the context of demands for money, at the constant risk of exposure to HIV, and have to shoulder the financial burden. In addition, women are accused by male family members of being responsible for drug misuse, of maintaining secrecy regarding the drug abuser, and of not getting timely treatment. Women most often become victims not just of drug abusers but also of the family and society at large.

Stigma and discrimination contribute tremendously to the spread of the virus. The focus of prevention strategies is on public health concerns, ignoring the fact that care and support to those already infected will serve not only to mitigate the impact of the disease on these individuals and their families, but to actually reduce the spread of the infection. Stigma also leads to denial of basic rights, including right to health care, housing, employment and education.

While all UN conventions and legal frameworks of most countries guarantee equal rights of women in all spheres, ground realities do not reflect these principles. Women are subjected to a range of derogatory practices and subjugation from the moment of conception to death, many of which further victimise women within the AIDS pandemic. These include sexual abuse, deprivation of matrimonial property, domestic violence and discrimination to name a few.

The legal system continues to perpetuate gender inequality and is ill-equipped to resolve difficulties faced by women in the social circumstances of HIV/AIDS particularly in the area of family issues, economic dependence, property rights, maintenance, custody of children, discrimination in health care, issues of consent and confidentiality, criminal law relating to harassment.

**Drawbacks of Mandatory Testing for HIV**

The fact that many women have got infected by their husbands has led many people and governments to believe that mandatory testing of couples prior to registration of marriage would help save the lives of many women. However, while all agree that voluntary testing should be encouraged, it is felt that mandatory testing would defeat the very purpose it aims to achieve, *viz.* reduction in HIV transmission to women and possibly children, apart from encroaching on the human rights of people. Some of the reasons against mandatory testing are:

- Mandatory testing violates privacy and confidentiality; people will be victimised and blamed, social divisions will be perpetuated.
- The 'window period' may eliminate people who are infected.
- Mandatory testing does not ensure behaviour change; risky sexual behaviour could continue after marriage.
- Marriages cancelled due to a person's HIV+ status will lead to victimisation and social ostracism of the entire family. Further, it is more than likely that people 'forcefully prohibited' from getting married as well as ostracised from their communities will have multiple sex partners.
- Mandatory testing is highly expensive both in human and financial terms and a burden on the health infrastructure.
- It is easy to obtain false reports for those who know their status and wish to get married anyway.
- People can resort to anti-retroviral therapy which could bring down the viral load to undetectable levels; this would ensure that the test results are seronegative.

The law also does not acknowledge women's primary role as carers, a role reinforced and perpetuated by society and extremely demanding due to the AIDS pandemic. Laws of inheritance, property, divorce and separation and custodianship of minor children are favourable to men. Nor is there prohibition under the law for non-consensual sex within marriage, which makes it difficult for women to refuse sex even if the husband is HIV+.

Health budgets are a political decision. Unfortunately, health is given increasingly low priority in National Health budgets the world over. Following current economic orhtodoxy, governments find themselves pressured into letting the private sector play an increasingly important role in health care and protection. This means that poorer sections of society are increasingly deprived of these services. In an already deprived access scenario, women get further marginalised

**Socio-Economic**

Women are denied access to income and property and have very little control over the family income. The responsibility for the care of the family however lies with women. The lack of viable economic choices often forces women into prostitution exposing them to a high risk of HIV infection. Women's control over their sexual and reproductive health is highly compromised given the gender inequalities within and without the family. Decisions to seek treatment for illnesses also lie with the purported 'head of the family'.

The socio-economic impact on women has further implications if one examines the trends of the epidemic. It is usually men who get infected and pass on the infection to their wives. HIV+ status is most often detected once the man is in the AIDS stage. The women is placed in a situation where she has to deal with her husband's illness and death, her resentments towards him for putting her in this situation, the responsibility of caring for him, her in-laws accusations that it is her 'fault', the possible denial of her property rights after his death and the financial insecurities and lack of economic alternatives. Her low financial status also has tremendous implications on her basic health and nutrition requirements further adding to her depression. The low status of a widow in our society further exacerbates an already traumatic situation.

In some cases women do gain support from the family and society particularly when the husband's lifestyles were publicly known—multiple sexual partners, drug or alcohol abuse etc. However, even in these cases, the woman is made to feel obliged for the support and sympathy that she is receiving and her fears about who will look after her in her last days continue to be very real.

The impact of HIV/AIDS on poverty, gender and the economy, and the interplay of factors like conflict and violence further increase gender linked vulnerabilities to HIV/AIDS. Not only does HIV thrive in an environment of poverty, it deepens existing poverty and inequality. As majority of the people infected are in the productive and re-productive age group, the pandemic has reversed much of the economic progress that has taken place in some countries. Further, due to the lack of access to information, education and health services, it is the already marginalised and poorer sections of the society who are the most severely affected. Cut-backs in education, welfare and health provisions have affected the poor the most. Dwindling employment opportunities reduce the economic choices that people have. Migration to urban areas is common and as women often lack the education or skills to get formal employment, often their only choice is commercial sex work. Even in cases where they find other means of employment, sexual abuse by employers is extremely common.

According to a recent report by the UN's World Food Programme, food is the primary concern for the families of people living with HIV/AIDS in majority of the developing countries. When the family's breadwinner becomes ill, families are often forced to sell off productive assets, spend their savings on food and medicine, and withdraw children from school to put them to work or to care for sick adults. The report states that "Food consumption has been shown to drop by as much as 40 per cent in households affected by HIV/AIDS." Typically, it is the female-headed households that are the most vulnerable. In many parts of sub-Saharan Africa, women who have their own children often have the added burden of looking after the children of dead relatives and friends.

## Conflict and Violence

"Violence against girls and women causes more deaths globally among females aged 15 to 44 than traffic accidents, malaria, cancer or war." Gender based violence increases the vulnerability to HIV infection both directly and indirectly. In the former case, forced sex or rape as mentioned earlier increases the risk of infection due to torn tissues and exchange of blood. Indirectly, an atmosphere of violence does not allow for safe sex negotiations. In times of conflict and displacement girls and women are far more vulnerable. For one, they become victims of rape, which is used as an assertion of power and force during war times. The chances of getting infected is much higher as STI rates among soldiers, even in times of peace, are much higher as compared to civilians.

In the increasing scenario of violence due to terrorism, communalism, racism and so on, power is sought to be obtained through violence. From Rwanda to Gujarat, one can see how women are the worst sufferers and in the growing AIDS pandemic, at the greatest risk of getting infected.

In Goa, while all the above factors have a role to play in increasing women's vulnerability to HIV/AIDS, there are certain specific peculiarities of the Goan situation. The long history of colonial rule has left a legacy of westernisation with its package of certain permissive lifestyles. These go along with traditional cultures where speaking about these issues leave alone acknowledging them are taboo. The flourishing tourist trade has increased acceptability of multiple sexual relations and those that go beyond the bounds of what are considered traditional social structures. All this is further attentuated by the economic and political decisions to increase the tourist trade at tremendous social costs. Goa is thus portrayed as a land of wine, women and song.

Further, Goa has the distinction of hosting one of the country's few clearly organised and demarcated red-light areas, frequented by locals and tourists alike. Apart from the red-light area there is a lot of commercial sexual activity along the beaches, part of the price society pays towards making Goa a tourist state.

There is also a high incidence of migration, both by labourers from neighbouring states and by locals to other states/countries. In both cases, it is most often the men who migrate leaving their wives and children behind. The long periods of separation provide grounds for extra-marital relationships.

Efforts are being made globally and locally to address the concerns of women's vulnerability ranging from policy statements at the Beijing Conference in 1995 and the declaration at the UN General Assembly Special Session (UNGASS) on HIV/AIDS in June 2001 to micro-level interventions at the local and regional levels. Let us look at some of the progress made towards addressing gender concerns.

The Platform for Action, Fourth World Conference on Women, Beijing, 1995 also deals with issues concerning women in the HIV/AIDS context. Para 98 states that women 'often do not have the power to insist on safe and responsible sex practices and have little access to information and services for prevention and treatment .... The social, developmental and health consequences of HIV/AIDS and other sexually transmitted diseases need to be seen from a gender perspective'. Strategic Objective C3 contains an extensive list of actions to be taken, including 'Developing gender-sensitive multi-sectoral programmes and strategies to end social subordination of women and girls and to ensure their social and economic empowerment and equality; facilitate promotion of programes to educate and enable men to assume their responsibilities to prevent HIV/AIDS and other sexually transmitted diseases.

The Second International Consultation on HIV/AIDS and Human Rights, Geneva, September 1996, recommended guidelines for implementation by the States in order to promote and protect human rights in the context of HIV/AIDS. These guidelines focus on activities by States in view of their obligations under international and regional human rights instruments. Guideline 8 refers to `women, children and other vulnerable groups' It says that 'States should, in collaboration with and through the community, promote a supportive and enabling environment for women, children and other vulnerable groups by addressing underlying prejudices and inequalities through community dialogue, specially designed social and health services and support to community groups.'

Political commitment has had demonstrable effects on the curbing the spread of HIV. The UN Millenium Summit of September 2000 created the Millenium Development Goals, which included a commitment to halt and begin to reverse the global spread of the pandemic by 2015. One of its specific goals is to "promote gender equality and empower women".

The political momentum to deal with the pandemic at the global level culminated in June 2001 when all the members of the United Nations met in a Special Session of the General Assembly to agree on a comprehensive and global response to the AIDS crisis. The Declaration of Commitment made by the Special Session and adopted unanimously serves as a benchmark for global action. One of its targets and goals is to "empower women as an essential part of reducing vulnerability to HIV". More specifically, paragraph 61 states "By 2005, ensure development and accelerated implementation of national strategies for women's empowerment, promotion and protection of women's full enjoyment of all human rights and reduction of their vulnerability to HIV/AIDS through the elimination of all forms of discrimination as well as all forms of violence against women and girls." Other goals though not directly emphasising gender concerns, reflect these in their implementation. More importantly, the Declaration, which is grounded in respect for human rights has served to define agendas and create a common platform for action. Measurements of progress towards the targets established at the UNGASS, for instance, reflect a need to significantly increase women's access to HIV testing in order to meet targeted reductions in the proportion of infants infected with HIV.

***UNGASS Goals***

- Stressing that gender equality and the empowerment of women are fundamental elements in the reduction of vulnerability of women and girls to HIV/AIDS.
- Challenging gender stereotypes, attitudes and inequalities regarding HIV.
- Implementing measures to increase women's capacity to self-protect.
- Eliminating all forms of violence against women to reduce vulnerability to HIV.

The Convention on the Elimination of All Forms of Discrimination Against Women (CEDAW) embodies human rights concerns which have special relevance within the HIV/AIDS context. It particularly deals with inequality in relation to health services, education, family relations, employment, violence against women, stereotypes and harmful cultural practices, child bearing, rural women and political representation.

Finally, the most recent attempt to ensure gender concerns become integral in our dealing with the pandemic has been the development of "Women and HIV/AIDS: The Barcelona Bill of Rights" This is a global effort initiated by Women at Barcelona and Mujeres Adelante with lead involvement by the International Women's AIDS Caucus of the International AIDS Society and the International Community of Women Living with HIV/AIDS. Women and girls from around the world are called upon to unite to declare our rights and urge all governments, organizations, agencies, donors, communities and individuals to make our rights a reality.

Policy documents, declarations and statements would be meaningless if not translated into strategies and programmes that are implemented. Efforts are being made by international agencies, national governments, NGOs and civil society to reduce gender-linked vulnerabilities in the AIDS context.

Most of the international agencies have separate programmes to address gender issues, while attempting to integrate gender in the other programmes as well. Gender issues have become an important component of training programmes on HIV/AIDS across the world.

The Indian Government, through the National AIDS Control Programme attempts to address gender concerns through priority general interventions and through the targeted intervention programmes. While the first deals with specific needs and vulnerabilities of the general population, the latter focuses on highly vulnerable populations like commercial sex workers, men who have sex with men, migrant populations, street children etc. Within these programmes, there are attempts to address causes of women's vulnerability and reduce gender imbalances.

There is now a specific programme to Prevent Mother-to-Child Transmission (PMTCT) programme. For some years now, it has been well established that ground breaking progress has been made in preventing infants from getting infected. In Africa, MTCT programmes including anti-retroviral therapy, have proven to be highly effective in preventing the transmission of HIV to new-borns. However, the absence of care for mothers is only recently being recognised and attempts to integrate this care are underway. It is unfortunate that this need is being felt more due to the disincentive that women have to participate in the programme rather than as a moral issue.

However, a lot of the concerns shown for women in the HIV/AIDS context have questionnable motives. Preventive strategies, which primarily target commercial sex workers, stem from concerns about public health rather than the individual women infected and affected.

Moreover, gender is still an add-on to many programmes and has not become completely integrated into the mainstream HIV/AIDS programme. Nor do some of the programmes specifically for women seek to address root causes of vulnerability like poverty, gender relations within the society and family, socio-cultural concerns and so on. The PMTCT programme is one such example.

Within these programmes at the implementation level the inclusion of gender concerns is rather cosmetic in nature since the programme managers and the staff responsible for implementation often do not have genuine concern for these issues.

A lot, therefore, remains to be done, which includes efforts by governments, multilateral agencies and donors to put in place social protection and safety nets for people hardest hit by the pandemic, enhancing an understanding of gender relations and roles and the spread of HIV, translating policy statements into interventions, incorporating gender analysis into HIV/AIDS work at the community level, inter-sectoral collaboration and integrating rights-based frameworks to address root causes of vulnerabilities.

### *Some of the Specific Ways We Could Work Towards more Effectively Incorporating Gender Concerns and Reducing the Vulnerability of Women are Mentioned Below*

It is essential to integrate human rights with public health principles in HIV prevention. An effective community development approach to HIV/STI prevention must make community participation real by: building human and community capacity to participate, creating the social space for participation, and transferring project ownership to the community.

There is a need to place the PMTCT programme as a part of other services. The programme as envisaged is very medical-centred. It needs to include other disciplines as well the general community. Also, it reinforces the emphasis on the role of women as mothers. What about other women?

HIV interventions should incorporate the social context in which they operate. Gender norms often sanction violent expressions of husbands' locus of control in the household. As women try to minimize exposure to violence, their ability to insist on monogamy, negotiate condom use or refuse sex is limited. Prevention campaigns targeting men rather than women may effectively reduce women's risk of HIV.

Men also need to be engaged as partners in AIDS prevention and care, particularly in places where they are key decision-makers in matters related to health care.

STI/HIV prevention efforts need to be a part of a larger process of empowering women in which there is a discussion of reproductive, sexual and health rights. This is because gender inequalities, manifested in a variety of ways, have resulted in women accepting extremely high thresholds of suffering and not seeking timely treatment for their symptoms.

There is an urgent need to reform laws affecting women, and to empower women by providing a strong system of structural legal support. It is also imperative that personal law reform be undertaken with a particular view to meeting the gender-specific needs of women infected and affected by HIV/AIDS.

Mere awareness and behaviour change communication is insufficient if deep-rooted gender-based vulnerabilities are ignored. Prevention programmes need to adopt an integrated gender perspective addressing power relations within relevant socio-cultural and economic contexts.

Women's access to information, education, income-generating opportunities and health services including appropriate and ethical HIV testing and counselling needs to be increased.

There is an urgency to stimulate political will across the board to address issues like stigma and discrimination and make care and support concerns an integral part of prevention programmes.

International agencies, national governments, local NGOs and civil society need to understand and acknowledge the linkages between development, gender and HIV/AIDS. There is a need to create stronger international cooperation at all levels.

Existing strategies and programmes should be modified taking into consideration gender based realities.

A more equitable distribution of resources would go a long way in increasing women's access to services thereby reducing their vulnerability both to HIV infection and AIDS.

Issues of poverty, food security, adequate water supply would need to be addressed, particularly in developing countries. These issues also need to be integrated in the existing programmes.

National Health Policies and others exclude women and/or HIV+ persons. The various government schemes should not be seen in isolation, but incorporated into the HIV/AIDS programme.

It is well accepted that across the world, it is women who shoulder the entire responsibility of providing care and support. It cannot be argued that this has a massive cost—to women personally, to children and families, to women's ability to work and earn an income, to their ability to participate in social and political processes at the community and other levels. We need to categorically recognise the economic and social contribution of this care burden that women bear. Where possible financial compensation must be given and the rights and status of women in society must be urgently improved.

In order to ensure better access national capabilities to deal with the epidemic need to be strengthened particularly to safeguard the right to health. This would include improved health infrastructure, provision of various facilities for testing, counselling and treatment, development of vaccines and so on. It would be beneficial to involve the business sector in these efforts and integrate this sector in the entire AIDS programme.

An essential part of enabling environment involves the empowerment of women and other vulnerable sections of the community by improving their social and legal status in order to deal with HIV/AIDS. Women have to be involved in the design and implementation of programmes.

Health programmes should integrate gender sensitive HIV/AIDS components like HIV prevention, voluntary counselling and testing and STD management.

Where community based organisations and NGOs have begun the process of creating a supportive and enabling environment to reduce women's vulnerability to HIV/AIDS, governments must recognise these efforts and lend legal, financial and political support to strengthen them.

Women and women's organisations need to be included in HIV/AIDS policy development, strategizing, programming and implementation at all levels.

Governments, especially when they sign or ratify conventions, should be held accountable to their countries to ensure that commitments made are fulfilled. NGOs are in an ideal position to hold governments to account through advocacy campaigns. We need to generate greater accountability and transparency of international agencies and institutions.

Gender-based indicators need to be developed for monitoring the progress of programmes and strategies.

## Conclusion

In the final analysis, attempts to reduce gender-linked vulnerabilities in the HIV/AIDS context will only be effective if programmes take into consideration the various ways in which power imbalances between women and men and reflected at various levels and dimensions impact on women.

> I will conclude with a quote by Cindy Berman, of ILO
>
> "We cannot any longer continue to talk about home and community based care without addressing the roles and responsibilities of governments to provide adequate social protection and social services. We can no longer talk about workplace policies without examining the gender impact of care burdens, and how women are effectively excluded from decent work opportunities—whether formal or informal work because there is no-one else to care for the sick and dying in their homes and communities.
> We can no longer talk about support for AIDS orphans without putting in place mechanisms to ensure that children can go to school free of charge and have the opportunities to learn skills, avoid exploitative child labour, and be able to contribute to the economy and society with an education and

opportunities for decent work. We can no longer talk about project development without including the care economy and gender dimensions of poverty—not in a tokenistic way, but in a way that addresses the reality of people's daily struggle for survival, and the urgent need for social safety nets."

## REFERENCES


Action, Aid, ACORD and Save the Children (2002): *Gender and HIV/AIDS: Guidelines for Integrating a Gender Focus into NGO Work on HIV/AIDS,* Save the Children, London.

Bandopadhyay, N. *et al.,* (2002): 'Operationalizing an Effective Community Development Intervention for Reducing HIV Vulnerability in Female Sex Work: Lessons Learned from the Sonagachi Project in Kolkata, India', Paper presented at XIV International AIDS Conference, Barcelona.

Dale, Penny (2002): *As Hunger Stalks Southern Africa, HIV/AIDS is the Price Women Pay,* Inter Press Service.

Dubey, N. (2002): 'Indian Laws Exacerbate the Vulnerability of Women to HIV', Paper presented at XIV International AIDS Conference, Barcelona.

*Global Burden of Disease, Harvard University, 1996, cited in* Heise, L., Pitanguy, J., and Germain, A. (1994), 'Violence Against Women: The Hidden Health Burden', World Bank Discussion Paper 255.

Global Health Council, MTCT-plus: *Spearheading HIV/AIDS Prevention and Care for Mothers and Children,* Global Health Council.

Go, V.F. *et al.,* (2002): 'Marital Violence in India: Women's Heightened Vulnerability to HIV/AIDS', Paper presented at XIV International AIDS Conference, Barcelona.

International Council of AIDS Service Organisations (2002): *HIV/AIDS and Human Rights,* International Council of AIDS Service Organisations, Toronto.

International Council of AIDS Service Organisations (2002): *Update on the UNGASS Declaration of Commitment on HIV/AIDS,* International Council of AIDS Service Organisations, Toronto.

Kumar, Sanjay (2002): *Women and Drug Abuse: The Problem in India,* report published by United Nations International Drug Control Programme and India's Ministry of Social Justice and Empowerment.

Thomas, C. (1996): 'Global Burden of the HIV Pandemic', *The Lancet,* Vol. 248, July 3: 99-106.

United Nations (1998), *HIV/AIDS and Human Rights - International Guidelines,* New York and Geneva.

UNAIDS (2001): *Statistical Charts – UNAIDS (2001) :AIDS Epidemic Update December 2001.*

United Nations Development Fund for Women (2001): *Turning the Tide: CEDAW and the Gender Dimensions of the HIV/AIDS Pandemic,* UNIFEM, New York.

World Health Organisation (2002): *Scaling Up the Response to Infectious Diseases: Report on Infectious Diseases 2002,* WHO, Geneva.

For Barcelona Bill of Rights see website: http://archives.healthdev.net/gender-aids.

For Declaration of Commitment to Combating HIV/AIDS 2001 see www.unaids.org/ whatnew/others/un_special/declaration020801_en. htm

For Platform for Action and the Beijing Declaration from the Fourth World Conference on Women, Beijing, 1995 see www.un.org/womenwatch/daw/beijing/platform.

Data from GSACS and Department of Microbiology, Goa Medical College.

# 10

# SEX EDUCATION

## A Different Perspective

*Sheela Gupte*

The arrival of HIV and AIDS at out own doorstep has brought about a dramatic change in the field of sex education for adolescents. The reluctance or even frank opposition that characterised the attitude of most parents and teachers to this issue has disappeared. Today, many schools, colleges and other institutions demand sex education programmes; and there are several NGOs, private individuals and Government agencies that are involved in providing such education. The contents of almost all such programmes, at least in India, are based on the premise that providing accurate information to adolescents about sexual matters will result in a desirable change in their attitude and that, this, in turn, will bring about appropriate modifications in their behaviour. This paper seeks to examine these assumptions or hopes.

Despite the conflicting opinions regarding the content of sex education programmes, everyone agrees that its final aim is to bring about a reduction in risky sexual behaviour, the risks being unwanted pregnancies and sexually transmitted diseases, including HIV/AIDS and probably also some forms of cervical cancer. It would have been easy to examine the effectiveness of present educational programmes if sufficient number of well-designed controlled studies were available to see if adolescent behaviour did change as a result of such programmes. However, I am not aware of any significant studies in India which have specifically focused on the impact of existing sex education programmes on actual risky sexual behaviour, as opposed to their impact on levels of information. Given the paucity of such data in our country, we need to look at other ways to try and address this question.

As a practising gynaecologist, I see several adolescents who have actually got into trouble with unwanted pregnancies or STD's. Almost none of these teenagers were actually uninformed about the consequences of their actions. Most of them knew very well that sexual intercourse can lead to pregnancy and that some diseases are sexually transmitted. Quite a few teens today also know about AIDS. I agree that they may be ignorant or have misconceptions about many of the details. But after all, one does not need to know the technical details about ovulation, menstruation, fertilisation etc. to know that sexual intercourse can result in a pregnancy. Similarly one does not need to know the correct names of the different STD's, or the exact chances of getting infected to be aware that some serious diseases can be transmitted sexually.

The point is that, in spite of being aware of the risks that they were taking, they did take those risks. The question is, why?

Is a teenage boy who speeds by on a motorcycle not aware of the risks of dangerous driving? He knows that speeding can cause him to crash and he has very sure knowledge of the possibility of losing his life or limb. There is no secrecy or sense of shame involved in the transmission of knowledge about the risks of such driving. The 'culture of silence' which surrounds issues concerning sex is not applicable here, and yet we see some adolescents driving dangerously. Clearly, the reasons for risk-taking go beyond mere lack of accurate of information.

If any more proof were needed to convince us that it is not just lack of information that makes any individual take sexual risks, witness the number of urban, married, educated adults who end up with unwanted pregnancies or STDs. Surely neither lack of knowledge, nor lack of availability of protective measures, nor embarrassment at procuring these measures are at work among these educated urban elite. If some so-called responsible adult can engage in such sexual risks, we certainly need to look at more complex factors that can cause adolescents to take similar risks.

Many studies have found that sexual risk-taking is usually not an isolated form of risk-taking but is rather a part of multiple risk-taking behaviour.

Based on the insights which I have gained from my clinical practice, I wish to propose that :

1. It is likely that efforts made to tackle risk taking behaviour in general might yield more dividends in terms of reduced rates of STDs and unwanted pregnancies.
2. Existing sex education programmes need to be modified if we wish to go beyond mere dissemination of information and aim to reduce sexual risk-taking.

With this in mind, I take a closer look at risk behaviour.

**Risk-Taking**

Risk behaviour during teenage has been defined as voluntary behaviour that threatens the well-being of teens and limits their potential for achieving responsible adulthood. The dividing line between the normal exploratory behaviour, which is part of adolescence, and risk-taking behaviour could be hazy.

Some of the risky behaviours that have been identified are:

Alcohol use (both regular and binge drinking), tobacco use, other illegal drug use, fighting, weapon carrying, suicidal thoughts and attempts, risky sexual activity, dangerous driving, eating disorders and criminal activity. Patterns of risky behaviour are changing and perhaps cyber crimes could be added.

Several factors have been identified which might lead to or have been associated with general risk taking behaviour in adolescents. These are:

*Risk Taking as an Expression of Rebellion*

Rebelliousness is part of the natural process of growing up. It is the process by which teenagers try to establish their independent identity. But when such acts of rebellion threaten their own short or long-term well-being—it can be termed as risky behaviour.

(Here is what some teenagers who have indulged in risky behaviour have to say about why they did it—"My parents don't understand me" "Life sucks".)

*Peer Pressure*

Young people have a great tendency to conform to the norm that they perceive among their peers. They hate or dread being different from what they perceive their contemporaries to be.

*Denial*

Even adults can be victims of denial, but teenagers are especially prone to believe that they themselves are immune to the risks they know they are taking. They have a strong sense of personal invulnerability. A teenager is likely to say, "Nothing bad will happen to me—look at the odds—the risks are only 2 in 100".

*Alcohol Abuse*

It is easy to understand how the use of alcohol contributes to every kind of risky behaviour by clouding judgement when a person is drunk. Apart from this, even the history of alcohol abuse either by the teenager himself or in his family could be an indicator or marker that the teen may be prone to risk-taking behaviour.

*Other Social Factors*

Research has linked adolescent risk-taking behaviour to broken families, absent parents, low income families, low level of father's education, alcohol abuse in the family, very permissive parenting, low school grades, lack of belief in a bright future etc.

In 1995, the U.N. Fourth World Conference on Women, which met in Beijing, declared that "contrary to popular belief, adolescence is a time when many young people continue to need parental attention. Parental support can provide powerful protection against the possibility that they may engage in unhealthy practices, become socially isolated or become troubled or depressed".

The National Longitudinal Study of Adolescent Health found that "teenagers with strong emotional attachment to their parents and teachers are much less likely to use drugs and alcohol, attempt suicide, engage in violence, or become sexually active at an early age".

## Sexual Risk-Taking

Having said that sexual risk taking is usually part of a general tendency to take risks, it must be admitted that certain factors also determine sexual risk-taking in particular. These are:

- The biological factor.
- Low self-esteem.
- History of sexual or physical abuse.
- Subconscious wish to get pregnant.
- Conscious desire to get pregnant.
- Trivialisation of the MTP procedure.

*The Biological Factor*

The human species must be unique in that in a human, the awakening of sexual maturation does not coincide with psychological or developmental maturity or even financial stability, which are requisites for starting a family. Thus adolescents are caught in a situation where they are " high on hormones, but low on judgement" It must be realised that the sexual drive is a strong innate biological urge and that the general risk-taking behaviour of an adolescent can easily manifest as sexual risk-taking.

*Low Self-Esteem*

Actually this may contribute to general risk-taking, but is very striking in teenagers taking sexual risks. Adolescents, especially girls, have an overwhelming desire to please. The approval of another person, especially a member of the opposite sex, makes them feel they are complete. The lower the person is in self-esteem, the higher the likelihood that he or she will measure his or her completeness by the degree of the approval of others. Teenagers or even adults do not often realise that relationships based merely on a desire to please and earn the approval of the other are not happy in the long run.

So, having sex or not being able to say no to sex is often a teenager's way of re-assuring himself or herself of his/her own worth.

> "I had sex because my boy friend wanted it so much, besides he said he would be permanently damaged if I did not let him".
> "He needed me so much, it made me feel very important".
> "He made me feel attractive".

*History of Sexual or Physical Abuse*

While it is clear that forced sexual intercourse may directly result in pregnancy, the path by which sexual abuse at a young age leads to high-risk behaviour is less direct. Premature, exploitative and coercive sexual experiences may form the socio-emotional contexts of such behaviour. Possible consequences of childhood sexual abuse are promiscuity and the self-perception of being promiscuous, low self-esteem and decreased locus of control.

### *A Subconscious Wish to Get Pregnant*

It is said that humans have a need to know that they are fertile, which does not necessarily mean that they want a child. Part of the depression that men and women sometimes suffer from, after undergoing surgical sterilization is attributed to their knowledge that they are no longer fertile. It is hypothesized that some teenagers who get pregnant and especially those who get pregnant repeatedly, are being driven by the desire to prove their ability to conceive. Indeed many tribal cultures have institutionalised ways of proving a person's fertility before a marriage can be formalised.

### *A Conscious Desire to Get Pregnant*

This may arise from the mistaken belief that a pregnancy will cement a shaky relationship. Some teenagers seem to believe that a boy can be coerced into a marriage if they get pregnant. More often they are not, they end up precipitating the inevitable break up.

### *Trivialisation of the MTP Procedure*

A great deal of research and organised effort has gone into making safe abortions available to women in India. Unfortunately, however, there is a growing public perception that medical termination of pregnancy is a trivial procedure. Psychological morbidity apart, there are inherent risks involved in an MTP and it deserves to be taken more seriously. It seems probable that this trivialisation of MTP could have encouraged sexual risk-taking among adolescents and adults alike.

There is another aspect of this. An unwanted pregnancy is no longer the principal concern of sexual risk-taking. An unwanted pregnancy is treated as an easily curable disease. Our main concerns are STDs, notably, HIV/AIDS. If adolescents venture to take risks because they know that a pregnancy can be discretely terminated, forgetting that STDs are the main risk today, then they are living under a false sense of security.

## The Place of Present Sex Education Programmes

Teenagers have an intense desire and need to know more about sexual matters. They deserve access to accurate and reliable information. And this is what sex education programmes today aim to provide, which in itself is a valuable service.

Shireen Jeejebhoy, quoting a study in Gujarat, based on a system of obtaining anonymous questions through letter boxes placed in schools and colleges, says that "among girls, the major concerns in classes 7-8 is menstruation, by classes 9-12 it is physical appearance and only among college girls do issues of sexual relations become important. Among boys, the main interest in class 7-8 is in questions regarding normal sexual behaviour, nocturnal emission and male and female anatomy. By class 9-12 interest shifts to more specific and personal questions on masturbation, body size and condoms. Among college boys, questions pertain to mature adult sexual behaviour and sexual satisfaction".

Thus sex education programmes devised in culturally sensitive ways to address these concerns will go a long way in reducing anxieties and confusion and will hopefully prevent information being accessed from unreliable sources.

But let us not assume that this is sufficient to have any significant impact on risky sexual behaviour among teens.

## Some Problems with Present Sex Education Programmes

Several contradictions and inconsistencies beset present day sex education programmes. I will take up only the most glaring among them.

### *Diverse Messages*

In the West, there has been a considerable debate over what message to give to adolescents about preventing STDs and pregnancy. Lynn Blinn Pike, the Director of the Centre on Adolescent Sexuality, Pregnancy and Parenting at the

University of Missouri, Columbia, in an article in July 1999 summarised these conflicting messages as follows:

- Remain abstinent until marriage.
- Remain abstinent until emotionally and developmentally ready to be sexually active.
- Remain abstinent, but if not able to, have accurate and factual information about birth control and protections.
- Have accurate and factual information on how to use birth control and protection effectively, because abstinence is not a realistic expectation.

Such conflicting messages are confusing to youth. Here in India, we have had no comprehensive debate on what messages to give to the adolescents. There has been almost no community participation in this scanty discussion, except probably in church-based marriage formation courses.

In the absence of such a debate and reasonably uniform standards, sex education programmes run the risks of being irrelevant or worse still, inviting frank opposition from parents and teachers.

### Setting-up Expectations that Everybody is Doing It

Most sex education programmes are imparted in a manner, which subtly sets up the whole target group to assume that everybody of their age is having sex, which teenagers can misconstrue to mean that they are expected to be sexually active. The time devoted to those youth who abstain is far less than that devoted to early sexual activity and the risks thereof. Taken with the well-known tendency to conform to the perceived norms, we can imagine the potential for damage.

### Incorrect or Insufficient Information

Condoms are being touted as the ultimate defense against contracting the HIV through sexual intercourse. I do not know from where or how the effectivity of condoms in preventing

HIV transmission is being quoted as 99-100 per cent. Even as a contraceptive, and under ideal circumstances of condom use, *i.e.* use at each and every intercourse and no genital to genital contact without it, condoms are not 100 per cent effective. Incidents of accidental breakage and slippage are not uncommon even with experienced men within stable sexual relationships. Obviously, among adolescents, where sexual encounters usually occur "spontaneously and surreptitiously depending largely on opportunities for privacy" (Goparaju, 1993), even if condoms were made freely available, there is every reason to believe that they may not be correctly used, if used at all. Hence, in reality, the protection offered by the condoms may be far less than assumed.

On the other hand, an inexperienced adolescent boy who is armed with a condom might believe himself safe and therefore feel secure in taking risks. His sense of security is ill founded. As far as the adolescent girl is concerned, she is unlikely to have negotiating skills required to make a reluctant boy use a condom. So keeping a condom in her purse, which itself is unlikely, is not going to help much. The female condom is simply not available in India.

Other contraceptives, like the pill, are of course ineffective in preventing STDs. But adolescents who are using them might be encouraged to take risks knowing that they are protected against pregnancies, unmindful of the fact that they are thereby exposing themselves to higher risks of acquiring STDs.

The scientifically, factually correct statement would be that abstinence is the only 100 per cent effective way of preventing pregnancies and STDs and all protective measures offer varying degrees of protection against pregnancies but give either far less or no protection against STDs.

It is alright for the Government to promote condoms to reduce the rates of transmission of AIDS, because a fall by even a small percentage in the number of expected cases will result in a huge saving of costs. But is this enough protection for the individual adolescent?

**Results of Some Controlled Trials**

There are conflicting claims and counter claims regarding the positive effects of sex education.

It has been claimed that liberal sex education in Europe has succeeded in postponing teens' first sexual intercourse as compared to America. Upon closer inspection, the postponement appears to be by a few months, which prompted the Beijing Conference to declare that "the negative emotional and physical consequences of pre-marital sex are the same regardless of this age difference"

A very recent article in the *British Medical Journal,* June 2002 has published results from a systematic review of randomised controlled trials of interventions to reduce unintended pregnancies in adolescents.

The authors, Alba Dicenso, Gordan Guyatt, A. Willan and L. Griffin searched the available literature from 1970 to December 2000 and when all the relevant studies had been identified, the list was sent to experts to review for completeness. Twenty-six randomized controlled trials, which met the criteria for minimizing biases, were then selected. Data extraction and data analysis for these studies was done using stringent standard methods. Here are their conclusions—Primary preventive strategies evaluated to date do not delay the initiation of sexual intercourse, improve use of birth control among young men or women or reduce the number of pregnancies in young women.

**What Can Be Done**

In the debate over the most appropriate approaches to reduce adolescent high risk sexual behaviour, more emphasis has been placed on understanding adolescents who report that they have had sex than on understanding those who have remained abstinent.

Lynn Blinn Pike, in an article in Family Relation, 1999, speaks of the need to design different preventive strategies to build protective factors that result in 'sexual resilience' in target groups of adolescents.

The concept of resilience was originally developed in the field of developmental psychology. In 1993, it was first used to understand adolescent sexual well-being. A sexually resilient youth can adapt successfully to and resist even the most challenging and threatening circumstances.

Blinn Pike says that sexually abstinent youth need to be helped to become sexually resilient because they face the same opportunities and pressures to have sex as their sexually active peers. He reported on a study conducted on about 700 students who had said that they had not any sex. He tried to identify the reasons why they had been abstinent. He found that the most frequent reasons for not having sex were—fear of AIDS, fear of becoming pregnant or getting someone pregnant, or fear of getting a disease. The moderately frequent reason was—believing that it is wrong to have sex before marriage. The least frequent reasons were—not knowing where to get birth control or protection, being embarrassed to use birth control or protection and not having enough money to buy birth control or protection. In his final analysis he found that:

1. Boys are more likely to cite fear-based reasons than girls.
2. Adolescents who drink are less likely to cite fear-based reasons than those who do not.
3. Adolescents who did not drink were significantly more likely to cite emotional reasons and conservative values than adolescents who drink.
4. Adolescents who did not use alcohol had better educated fathers, were from non-urban areas, had higher grades and were more likely to be living with both parents.

Based on these and other findings, the following recommendations are being made to promote sexual resilience on one hand and reduce sexual risk-taking on the other.

*1. Sending Concrete and Consistent Messages :* Two messages need to be sent throughout the community to build sexual resilience among youth. The first is that abstinence is the only 100 per cent effective way of preventing unwanted pregnancy and STDs. The second is a strong anti drinking message, since alcohol use is definitely related to undesirable sexual activity among youth.

2. *Counteracting the 'Everybody is Doing It' Myth with Facts:* The 'social norms model' approach tells us that young people's behaviour gravitates to the 'norm' they perceive. So a common perception that "everyone at school is having sex" may lead a youth to conclude "I guess, I will too, why be different?" A message that everybody is not doing it might help counteract false norms and imaginary peer pressure.

Gracy Andrews and Vikram Patel, reporting on a study from Goa titled 'Health Needs of Adolescents', say that only around 6 per cent of adolescents admitted that they had sexual intercourse. In subsequent Focus Group Discussion with teachers and students, it emerged that they believe this to be an understatement. In their estimate the figure should have been 15 to 30 per cent, which to me seems like a reasonably accurate estimate. This means that about 70 to 80 per cent of youth are not engaging in sexual activity. Emphasising this information will go a long way in counteracting the myth that everybody is doing it.

3. *Sharing Information on the Positive Benefits of Sexual Resilience :* There are a number of personal freedoms that result from abstinence. These include, freedom from fear of STDs and unwanted pregnancies, freedom to pursue educational and career goals, freedom to pursue relational skills without sexual pressure, freedom to pursue and maintain lifelong pair bonds, and freedom to deal with sexuality and its implications when one has more ego strength and perspective than one does in his teens. In fact, many teenagers in the West report a sense of relief on knowing that they are not expected to be sexually active.

4. *Parenting and Related Issues :* In the Focus Group Discussion already referred to, reported by Gracy Andrews and Vikram Patel, students observed that "adolescents indulge in sexual activity when neglected by parents or when they spend most of their time out of their homes or when proper information about sex is unavailable to them".

The U.N. Fourth World Conference held in Beijing in

1995, created a document called The Beijing Platform for Action, which declared that "a stable family facilitates greater parental involvement which fosters better relationships with youth". It also said that as more families become dual income or single parent, more and more of the young adolescent's time is unstructured and unsupervised, leading to risk-taking such as alcohol abuse or promiscuity. It declared that "strengthening two parent families and lessening financial burdens on them (thus hopefully reducing the need for dual income families) must be a priority when devising risk avoidance strategies for the girl child and all youth".

What we can do to encourage the stable two-parent family norm with ideal guidance from parents- neither too restrictive, nor too permissive—could be the subject of extensive debate and research, but it is definitely a nebulous and difficult task.

5. *Prevention of Abuse and Its Effects :* Students can be made aware of strategies to prevent physical and sexual abuse, self-defence and whom to turn to in case of abuse. Schools must adopt a zero-tolerance level for bullying and violence (Gracy Andrews and Vikram Patel). Identification of and counselling for those who have been victims in the past should be pursued actively.

6. *Improving Self-Esteem, Stress Management, and Negotiating Skills :* Parents and teachers can be sensitised to various ways of helping growing children to improve their self-esteem. Stress management and coping techniques can be taught within the family or through lectures and workshops.

7. *Guidance on How to Study and Career Guidance :* "Simple tips on how to manage time, for example, using time tables and how to identify weak areas and work on these, are important to help adolescents learn how to cope with their growing educational requirements. Information about career choices can be provided and counselling given in decision- making skills that would enable them to make informed career decisions (Gracy Andrews and Vikram Patel).

These two seemingly mundane recommendations can make very significant contributions by reducing school drop-out rates and improving self-esteem through better academic performance and more satisfying career choices. Their effect in reducing sexual risk taking may be more profound than that of the present sex education programmes.

## Conclusions

Existing sex-education programmes, with an emphasis on accurate and frank information, fulfil an important need of adolescents but are not enough to bring down rates of unwanted pregnancies and STD's among them.

Different programmes, which tell the truth about contraceptives and MTPs and incorporate negotiating skills need to be devised to help about 70 per cent of our adolescents who are sexually abstinent to become sexually resilient, and to avoid risky sexual experimentation.

For the group in which sexual risk-taking is part of general risk-taking behaviour, more profound measures like counselling for increasing self-esteem, strategies for stress management, coping techniques, dealing with physical or sexual abuse in the past etc. may be required.

But in the long run, general measures and policy decisions to encourage the stable two parent family norm with strong parental ties and values, discouraging the use of alcohol in the community, guidance on how to study and make career choices etc. will yield indirect but more convincing results.

## REFERENCES

Alba Dicenso, Gordon Guyatt, A. Willan and L. Grifith in June 2002 issue of the British Medical Journal.

Catherine Hurlburt reporting on the U.N. Fourth World Conference on Women held at Beijing in 1995.

Dewhurst- Textbook of Gynaecology for Postgraduates.

Gracy, Andrews and Vikram, Patel: Health Needs of Adolescents- A study from Goa.

Leena Abraham in Understanding Youth Sexuality- A Study of College Students in Mumbai.

Lynn Blinn-Pike, Director of Centre on Adolescent Sexuality, Pregnancy, and Parenting at University of Missouri, Columbia - July 1999 issue of Family Relations.

Shireen Jeejebhoy: Adolescent Sexual and Reproductive Behaviour- a review from the evidence from India.

# 11

# UNIVERSAL SCREENING FOR CERVICAL CANCER

## An Attainable Health Objective in Goa

*Eugene D'Silva* and *Pia Muriel Cardoso*

Invasive cancer of the cervix is the commonest Cancer affecting the female genital tract, and the second commonest Cancer in women. It afflicts women in the prime of their lives and has the highest incidence in the age range of 35-55. It results in reduced life expectancy of 15-20 years. Regrettably a majority of the cases diagnosed in India continue to be at advanced stages of the disease. Despite advances in treatment the prognosis remains dismally poor, with overall 5-year survival for all stages of the disease at 30-40 per cent.

World wide, invasive Cancer of the cervix is the second most common malignancy in women and the commonest genital Cancer; of the estimated 500,000 cases arising annually 77 per cent occur in developing countries (Parkin *et al.*, 1988). In many developed countries the introduction of an extensive, highly efficient population based screening programme, has resulted in a lower incidence of Cancer by 50-60 per cent and a reduced mortality from the disease by 80 per cent. The value of screening for cervical Cancer has been demonstrated beyond any reasonable doubt, by the experience of countries like Finland (Hakama, 1982). This has most certainly been achieved at an additional cost to the health care providers. This initial investment is more than offset by the cost of treating advanced disease, in addition to loss of productive life span. The accumulated evidence suggests that cervical Cancer is preventable and highly suitable for primary prevention. Awareness of the condition, education about the associated risk factors (such as sexually transmitted disease, smoking, promiscuity) coupled with effective cervical screening certainly reduces morbidity and mortality.

## National Perspective

The cervical Cancer burden in India alone has been estimated at 100,000/year in 2001 (Shanta *et al.*, 2000). The increasing HIV epidemic threatens to further exacerbate the incidence of Cancer of the cervix. In the absence of any control programme the incident number of Cancer cases is expected to be in the region of 140/100000, in many metropolitan cities. Regrettably, 70 per cent of the new cases continue to be at an advanced stage of disease at diagnosis, and despite advances in treatment the overall 5 year survival for all stages of the disease is dismally low with an average relative survival of 38.3 per cent (Nandakumar *et al.*, 1995).

## Medical Perspective

Current understanding of the epidemiology of the disease, suggests a gradual progression of pathology from a state of normality, through pre-Cancer cell change until the development of invasive Cancer, which takes between 7-10 years. The accessibility of the cervix to both cytological and clinical examination, coupled with the slow progression of pre-Cancer change offers the prospect for screening strategies to effectively prevent the development of invasive disease.

> Screening for cervical Cancer aims at identifying the women at risk for the disease, and treating those with pre-Cancer cell change, thereby reducing the incidence of cervical Cancer and the mortality from the disease.

It is almost certain that infection with some strains of the Human Papilloma Virus is a necessary prerequisite for the development of cancer of the cervix. This offers the exciting prospect of the development of a vaccine, which would control and eventually eradicate the disease. However until the development of such a vaccine, an organised universal-screening programme is the only means of reducing the morbidity and mortality associated with cervical Cancer.

*Cervical cytology remains the only viable method of screening for pre-Cancerous changes.* When abnormalities are detected on cytology, definitive diagnoses with histological confirmation is made using Colposcopy. Women in the age group of 20-60 are the targets of any cervical screening programme. This is because the incidence of invasive cancer in teenagers is rare (1 in 2 million) similarly there is a low incidence and mortality of cervical cancer after the age of 60. The interval between smears has great influence on the cost-effectiveness of any screening programme. Based on mathematical models the level of protection against the development of Cancer ranges from 64 per cent to 93 per cent depending on the frequency of the smears. (Day 1989) Even a single life time cytology screen offers protection against the disease of 10.2 per cent to 55.6 per cent (Agarwal *et al.*, 1995) depending at the age at which screening is done.

**Table 11.1:** Cervical Screening Programme

| *Frequency of screening in years* | *Protection against development of disease (in per cent)* |
|---|---|
| Smear every year | 93% |
| Smear every 3 years | 91% |
| Smear every 5 Years | 84% |
| Smear every 10 Years | 64% |
| Single Life time smear | 11-55% |

Current recommendations suggest that a woman whose smear shows either moderate to severe abnormality or persistent mild abnormality be referred for colposcopic assessment (Duncan, 1992).

The aim of Colposcopy is to detect pre-Cancerous disease and to then direct treatment, which is usually by local destructive or excisional methods, which can be safely performed under a local anaesthetic in an outpatient/office setting. The advantage of having histological confirmation on the completeness of treatment makes the excisional methods the preferred choice when dealing with higher-grade abnormality.

**State Perspective**

There is neither population-based data, nor hospital derived data available for the Cancer patterns in the state of Goa, and despite the National Cancer Registry Programme, there is no Cancer Registry existent in Goa. Significantly, cancer in general has received no attention in any of the health planning strategies of the State, although it remains the one of the leading five causes of death. The facilities for the comprehensive treatment of Cancers in the State of Goa are lamentably rudimentary and fractionated possibly because it is not seen as a major health concern and/or the lack of Specialist medical expertise in these areas. The establishment of a state level Cancer Registry and a move towards making Cancer a notifiable disease would highlight the extent of the problem, the mortality associated with it and would bring to fore the under-funding in this important area of Public Health.

With regard to cervical Cancer, it would be reasonable, in the absence of data, to assume that the trends would not be very different to that of the rest of the country. On the other hand, the financial and logistic constraints in the introduction and implementation of a National Cervical Screening Programme may not be applicable to the State of Goa. This is in view of its small size, high literacy, and health care infrastructure, which makes it ideal, for piloting a hospital-based cytological screening programme.

The resources required for the implementation of a successful and effective programme are low technology and reasonably cost effective, more so than many other areas of reproductive medicine. *Importantly the resources for smear collection, cytological evaluation and even Colposcopy are all available in Goa today and are underutilised mainly because of the lack of organised screening service.*

One of the most important parameters in any screening programme, is the coverage of the target population, which in the case of cytological screening would be women in the age group of 20-60. The level of coverage at the present time is very poor as can be seen from the data derived from the Goa Medical College for 2001.

**Table 11.2 :** Results of PAP Smears at GMC 2001

| | |
|---|---|
| Total Gynaecology attendance OPD | 12108 |
| Total No. Smears collected | 1201 |
| Total Normal Smears | 1173 |
| Dysplasia ( Abnormal -Pre-Cancer) | 21 |
| Malignant ( Cancer ) | 7 |

From the data available from countries where effective screening has come to stay, that the between 5-8 per cent of the smears would be expected to be reported abnormal if more than 85 per cent of the population of the target population was covered. If this were extrapolated to the above figures it would mean we should be seeing 280 cases of Invasive cancers and 840 cases of pre-Cancer in Goa Medical College alone if 85 per cent of the population attending the clinics were screened more diligently! This expected caseload corroborates well with the figures reported from the various registries in the country.

From the above discussions it is clear that, Invasive Cancer of the Cervix is a significant medical problem afflicting young women in the prime of their lives. The State of Goa has the resources, in terms of medical infra structure, human resource and technology to set up an effective screening programme for early diagnosis and treatment of pre-Cancer.

There can be no doubt that this would be at an additional cost to the health care system, especially in its initiation. However, it would be more than be balanced by the loss of productive years and the cost of treatment of invasive disease, notwithstanding the pain and suffering associated with the disease, for both the individual and family.

## Conclusion

I would like to emphasise that the whole objective of this paper was to bring to fore the problem of Cancer in Goa, and the lack organised strategies for prevention, early diagnosis and in many Cancers adequate treatment. I would be grateful if this audience would take home and reflect over the following concluding thoughts.

- Cancer of the cervix is a major health issue in women in their prime.
- Current understanding of the disease suggests that it is preventable.
- Cytological screening with Colposcopic assessment is a cost effective way of diagnosing and treating pre-Cancers even before women have symptoms.
- Cytological screening used effectively can reduce the incidence and mortality dramatically.

Importantly for us here in Goa

- There is a urgent need for establishment of State and Hospital based Cancer Registries, and consideration be given to making Cancer a notifiable disease.
- It is important to raise the profile of Cancer, because a large number of the common cancers are amenable to preventive strategies.
- Cancer should be at the core rather than the periphery of health planning for the future, because increased life expectancy, changing life styles, and the control of infections, will make cancer one of the major health problems of tomorrow.

Cytological screening for the prevention of cervical cancer is certainly logistically feasible in Goa at an affordable cost to the government.

## REFERENCES

Agarwal, S.S. *et al.*, (1995): 'Evaluation Of Hospital Based Cytology Screening Programme for Reduction of Lifetime Risk of Cervical Cancer', *Neoplasma:* 42 (2) 93-6.

Day, N.E. (1989): 'Screening for Cancer of the Cervix', *Journal of Epidemiology and Community Health:* 43: 103-106

Duncan, I.D. (1992) Cervical Screening Programme: Guidelines for clinical practice and programme management.National Coordinating Network Oxford.

Hakama, M. (1982): 'Trends in the Incidence of Cervical Cancer in Nordic Countries', *Hemisphere:* 279-92.

Nanadakumar, A., Anantha, N. and Venugopal, T.C. ( 1995): 'Incidence, Mortality, and Survival in Cancer of the Cervix in Bangalore India'. *British Journal of Cancer:* 71(6) 1348-52

Parkin, D.M. (1988): 'Estimation of worldwide frequencies of sixteen major cancers in 1980', *International Journal of Cancer:* 41184-97.

Shanta, V. *et al.*, (2000): 'Epidemiology of Cancer of the Cervix Global and National Perspective', *Journal of the Indian Medical Association:* 98(2) 49-52.

# HEALTH AND HUMAN RIGHTS ISSUES

# 12

# TOWARDS A RIGHTS APPROACH TO WOMEN'S HEALTH

## In a Sick System

*Albertina Almeida*

What is a rights approach to health? Why a rights approach? This paper presents an overview of the experiences of Bailancho Saad as regards health care for women, which have been gained in the course of interacting with women from various sections of society. The paper attempts to highlight those rights of women that are violated or rights that women are deprived of, in their day to day lives. The paper above all stresses on the need for appropriate accountable mechanisms to enforce rights from a gender perspective and calls for Gender Impact Assessment and entrustment of monitoring health concerns from a gender perspective and specifically looking at the implications for women.

In 1986 when Bailancho Saad got started and ever since, we have been interacting with several women from different section of society. Our activities with women have been varied. We have campaigned against commercialisation of culture—beginning with the campaign against the commercialised Carnival parade, to the campaigns for regulation of sex determination and against sex pre-selection, to campaigns against the economic development policies of the Government. In this process, we have had occasion to analyse the development policy, the tourism promotion policy, the employment policies of successive Governments and to see how these impact on the health of women. We have been organising Workshops on dealing with violence against women (including for school going children) and more recently also for men, in various parts of Goa, rural and urban institutions. We have been supporting individual women who needed assistance in following up their individual cases of harassment. We have been supporting groups of women from particular localities opposing the neglect, deprivation or the direct or indirect destruction of their water sources. We have been supporting groups of women opposing the setting up of a bar in their locality or opposing the manner in which the liquor outlet, has been violating the rules. In this process, we have also had the occasion to look at forensic reports. We have been organising issue-based State-level Workshops on alcohol, sexual harassment in employment, Workshops towards policies for women, children. We have been organising Workshops for Women Sarpanchas and Panchas to equip them to be prepared for their responsibilities and also to learn about their experiences through their first steps in formal political power. We have also been involved with a targeted intervention AIDS prevention project for the migrant slum population pockets in Tiswadi and Bardez.

Given this background, how do we see a rights approach as advancing the cause of women's health?

We will begin by looking at various seemingly disjoint instances in the day-to-day lives of women, which otherwise seemingly have no bearing on women's health:

(Most names in the instances below have been changed to respect the confidentiality of the women).

- Sarita, has two sisters and observes that her father is hankering for a son who he sees as the only possibility of salvation. Sarita's mother is made to undergo a sex determination test and when it is found that the foetus is female, Sarita's mother is pressurised to undergo an abortion. This happens twice. This gives Sarita a feeling of rejection and she gets into a depression. For Sarita's mother, two abortions and so also the piercing of the amniotic sac for extracting the amniotic fluid are taking a toll on her health.

- Susan, the Headmistress of a prominent girl's school in the suburbs of Panaji, tells us the children are malnourished. She says that most children have either not had a breakfast at all or have not had a nutritious breakfast. Given Goa's boy-preference, this is indicative of both the class and gender biases that work to reduce proper nutritional possibilities for girl children.
- We hold a health camp for college students in Canacona. One student musters the courage to tell us that her grandmother gives her brother an egg because he is a boy. Slowly the others begin to speak up about the discrimination in nutrition.
- Geeta, Meena and Nina have problems with their periods. They either get severe pain at the time they get their periods or get irregular periods and are too shy to approach a doctor or to find ways of ascertaining the why of their pain. There is also a taboo in talking about reproductive health problems which is why they take recourse in two's and three's. When we organised a health camp with the help of some doctors from GMC, we noticed young girls coming gradually in two's and three's to consult the doctors. This reflects a need for a conducive atmosphere to access health care.
- Jamuna was fifteen years old, when her parents get her married off. She belongs to a migrant Indian family from outside Goa. Due to early marriage and the ensuing pregnancy, she is weak and has not had the opportunity to develop her mental and physical faculties well. Similarly, Mariawwa was also fifteen years old when she was introduced into prostitution by an agent who manages to lure her parents who are poor and have no money to bring up Mariawwa. Due to early sexual intercourse and pregnancies, her proper development is also affected.
- Afroz and her neighbours draw water from a well for their use. They have been using water from that well for years. Suddenly one day some neighbours talk of stomach

disorders and Afroz realises that there must be a common problem as her family members are also inflicted by the same disorder. They trace it to the well-water, which has suddenly turned unconsumable. They follow up with the Sanitary Inspector of the Health Department who gives them bleaching powder to put in the well as a disinfectant. This doesn't work. The inhabitants of that ward realise that even as they disinfect the well is getting contaminated again. They soon are able to zero in on the possible source of well-water contamination—either a toilet which is built very close to the well in violation of the requirements of law that it should not be built within so many metres from a water source, or due to the effluents from a bar in the locality, which have deliberately been dumped into the well to spite their anti-alcohol movement. They want to be sure about the exact source, though, so that their right to potable drinking water doesn't become a mirage. The reply from the Environmental Laboratory in the Health Department is vague. They express their inability to discern. We have a right to know, the women say, and technological advances should be availed of for these purposes and be accessible to these women.

- Talking of technological advances, new reproductive technologies are often invasive or taking women's bodies and health for granted. Many women who are pregnant, for instance, are now invariably made to undergo periodic ultrasound tests. To add to this, they are not even told why they have to undergo these tests. Besides taking the woman's body for granted, they are ignoring the woman's right to self-determination and autonomy.
- And yet another reproductive technology invasion. Maria has no children. She is keen to adopt a child as she loves children. But her husband insists that they must have a biological child by hook or by crook. So she resorts to reproductive technology by which she almost risks her life. Who cares? Social conditioning holds the day, at all levels from the smallest unit of the family to the larger unit of State Government.

- There is enmity between two groups in a village. One of the groups decides to settle scores by putting some poison (and declaring as such) in the well that the other group uses. This means a longer distance, of walking to the next well, for the women who have been traditionally the water-fetchers for their families. It is women who therefore bear the double brunt of squabbles, riot programme. Innumerable studies of riot-torn areas have shown that sexual violence is a regular component of the riot programme. If health of a peoples and more particularly of women is a genuine concern, the State has to show it by desisting from fascist conduct which is a source as well as a generator of situations which cause physical and mental stress and insecurity for women.
- Jaimala, Sandhya and Minaxi are constantly complaining of back aches. When asked what could be the source of the aches, they all unanimously attribute it to the sterilisation which they underwent at a sterilisation camp with little knowledge of the consequences or measures to be taken post-sterilisation. A clear case of uninformed consent taken for sterilisation to meet targets. Target-free approach now. Fine, but do women's responses figure anywhere in the monitoring indicators?
- Sumedha has not had a proper meal for days now. She just collapses when she goes to the market sometimes. She has been conditioned to eat last. Barely able to afford a meal worth its name, eating last means virtually eating a few morsels. There is less fish available. The available fish finds itself on the plates of the tourists first. They can afford to pay for it. She can't. Her family has a flat now as against the old mud house. They bought the flat out of the money that the builder gave them when he bought the family field. But she and her family members can't eat the flat, can they?
- Soraya reports that somebody is setting up a golf course in her locality. That the Government has put an end in the papers to acquire land for the purpose. The ground was an open space where she took her cattle for grazing. But in the eyes of the Government, that land is "barren" land.

Has the Government thought of the implications of this golf course for the health of those in its environs? Golf Courses elsewhere have meant percolation of the chemicals used on them into the locality's water sources. Where is the health impact assessment? For women who have been traditionally engaged in health care for the family, where is the regard for the lengthening of their work day besides the consequences for their health? Did the Government consult the women? Did it do a Gender Impact Assessment? But how does one hold them accountable for not engaging in responsible consultative processes?

- Maira works in a factory that poses certain health hazards. The factory has the potential of having effects on her health as a human being in general and more particular effects on her as a woman. But Maira is on contract work. Given her job insecurity, she cannot hazard talking about occupational health hazards or even raising questions about the possible health hazards. What then?
- Kshama and her family are displaced because their land is acquired for the purposes of dam construction. No one asked who needed the dam and at whose cost the dam was going to be built. That was bad enough. But the State even failed in setting up an effective rehabilitation plan. Because it never considered that women did the survival work, that they worked in the house and in the adjoining field for sustenance of the family including themselves. They have been rehabilitated with a house which is allotted to the man and a job in the family means a job for the man of the family. What happened about the woman's life? What happened about the organic food that they ate?
- The smokeless *chullah* scheme when started was ostensibly intended to address women's health concerns. It should have been a runaway success. It wasn't. Did anybody take into account the stakeholders' opinions and realities in fashioning those schemes?
- There were two reported cases of conviction of health care providers for molestation in recent months; there is a serious need to look at this matter at this stage itself as

women resort to health care providers for their health very rarely and if it is seen as being unsafe, it will further limit women's spaces to health-care.

One could go on and on with examples. The list is endless. The point we are trying to highlight is: That women's human rights to health are violated or not regarded. The human rights involved are primarily the right to life and liberty which includes the right to live with dignity and the right to self-determination and autonomy, the right to equality and the right to freedom of expression implicit in not seeking women's consent or informed consent.

So, through interacting with individual women or groups of women, interacting with women in opinion-forming or decision-making roles, or collectively analysing the situations before us, some concerns have emerged:

1. That all the above said rights are there on the book or more precisely in the Constitution of India, but are violated, sometimes directly by the State itself, or not given effect to by the State.
2. That while addressing the concerns of individual women or groups of women from a particular locality, there are both micro-issues and macro-issues which have an impact on women's health.
3. That there are no appropriate accountability mechanisms to make the rights of women easily accessible and enforceable.
4. That the rights of women are in many respects inextricably linked to the rights of various other marginalised sections of society.
5. That socio-economic and political factors are determinants of the health status of women and any policy or steps or mechanisms developed must consider this.
6. That globalisation, privatisation and unsustainable production are taking their toll on women's health; loss of employment, displacement from shelters and livelihoods, feminisation of poverty, food insecurity are all eating into women's health.

7. That on the one hand, the forces of fanaticism and fascism are having their bearing on women's health and, on the other hand, technological advances made in science are also going the patriarchal way.
8. Health data and statistics collection is not gender disaggregated. Macro-planning and policy making for women's health is, therefore, a difficult proposition without the same.
9. Development projects are visualised/sanctioned without taking into account women's views and the impacts of those projects on women.

A rights approach to women's health, therefore, calls for:

1. Preventing violations of the rights.
2. Ensuring redressal of women's grievances about rights violations.
3. Listening to women's voices on health.
4. Pro-active steps and political stands that ensure that enabling conditions for women's health rights are created that are backed up by legislation to that effect.
5. Accountable enforcement mechanisms to ensure all the above must therefore be in place.

Suggested accountability and enforcement mechanisms are:

1. Programmes to address food security must be developed by involving the people and specifically the women from the concerned communities; this would also hold for other programmes being developed.
2. Making Gender Impact Assessment mandatory ( towards this gender impact assessment indicators must be evolved through consultative processes) for all policies.
3. Making Health Impact Assessment mandatory for all Policies, Plans and Projects to be sanctioned by the Government (just like Environment Impact Assessment but not with the restriction of this only to certain projects as is the case under the Environment Protection Act).

4. Making an officer each in the Directorate of Health and Goa Medical College responsible for viewing all health programmes from the point of view of meeting the needs and concerns of woman and from the point of view of their impact on women.
5. Specifically providing for gender-disaggregated statistics and data collection.
6. Priority in budget allocation for health and particularly women's health and this includes reproductive health, but reproductive health is just one aspect.
7. Setting up of a State-level Human Rights Commission for effective redressal of rights violations.
8. Gender sensitisation of health personnel and for that matter all Government personnel including Government officers at all levels, which would include the rights adjudicators.
9. Backing up any commitments to the above with suitable legislation, including appropriate modifications in the Goa Public Health Act to that effect.
10. Ensuring that the social justice committees envisioned under the Panchayat Raj Act are duly constituted, which will serve as fora for articulating social concerns which would include health concerns emerging at the grassroots level so that the same can be duly taken up by the Committees with their respective Panchayats or at their village gram sabhas, which can in turn articulate these concerns at larger fora. Something on similar lines can be done by the Municipalities through the committees that they constitute. Gender sensitisation of these social justice committees can go a long way so that the said Committees are equipped to have an ear for gender concerns.
11. Devising monitoring mechanisms to ensuring that access to health care is universal and that women are not deprived of such access by virtue of their caste, economic or social status, age, sexual orientation, marital status, guardianlessness or any other criteria.
12. Ensuring that there is no indirect deprivation of access to health care because of the non-availability of requisite medicines in the Government hospitals and health centres.

# 13

# PRIVATISATION, MEDICAL ETHICS AND WOMEN'S HEALTH

## Exploring Linkages

*Laxmi Murthy*

In a liberalised economy, medical research is increasingly being carried out by private institutions—non-governmental organisations (NGOs), pharmaceutical companies, private colleges and independent research institutions. With the gains of such research translating directly into huge profits, as in the case of contraceptive research, assisted reproduction, or the Human Genome Project, the need to understand the implications of such research cannot be overstated. While not arguing for increased statism and bureaucratic control, creative and effective ways of checking the 'free-for-all' are vital. As our experience with various contraceptive technologies has shown, monitoring by independent bodies is all the more crucial, because issues relating to medical ethics, accountability and monitoring the quality of the clinical research far from being academic subjects, have direct implications for women's health, safety and well-being.

### The Case of Depo-Provera

The introduction of the injectable contraceptive Depo-Provera (brand name of Depo-medroxyprogesterone acetate or DMPA) into India is representative of several aspects of the impact of privatisation on women's health. In 1994, Depo-Provera was approved for private marketing in the country despite the fact that it had not gone through all the mandatory phases of clinical trial in India. At the time, a case filed by Stree Shakti Sanghatana, Saheli and other women's groups raising questions about the safety of Net En, another injectable contraceptive (similar in action to Depo-Provera) was still pending in the Supreme Court. The Drugs Controller General of India (DGCI), while justifying the introduction of Depo-Provera in the name of a liberalised economy, however gave marketing approval on condition that the manufacturers conduct a post marketing surveillance (PMS).

The PMS sponsored by Pharmacia-Upjohn, the manufacturers of Depo-Provera, is illustrative of the adverse impact on women's health of privately sponsored research. PMS conducted by the pharmaceutical company which directly stands to profit from the results of the research, raises serious doubts regarding "scientific objectivity" of the data collected and its analysis. A concern of most health groups that was well borne out by the nature and findings of the 'study'.

The study is by no means an 'extensive five-year-long study' as promoted by the manufacturers. The report, finalised in October, 1999 and made public in September, 2000, is based on data collected from 1079 subjects recruited between June, 1994 and December, 1997. Yet, closer scrutiny reveals that each woman user is studied only over five 3-monthly injections *i.e.* for a period of 15 months only. There is no logic for this, since the intended duration of Depo-Provera is as a spacing method for at least 2 to 3 years. Fifteen months is inadequate to assess long-term effects, and it is therefore unscientific to declare Depo-Provera 'safe' on the basis of such inadequate data.

It is important to remember that contraceptives are administered to young, healthy women, and therefore the benefit-risk assessment should differ from the risk-benefit assessment of a treatment for a disease. A serious lacuna of the study design is that the potential side-effect of loss of bone-density [osteoporosis] leading to weakening of bones and fractures has not been studied. This issue is of great significance in India where bone-density among women is already low.

Significantly, cancer risk has also not been studied, though long-term studies in other countries show that increased risk of breast cancer—especially in younger women—cannot be ruled out. Assessment of return of fertility has not been incorporated in the study design—a serious lacuna in a contraceptive being promoted as a spacing method. This is all the more important in a country where significant gains have not been made to control infant mortality. Similarly, the effect on progeny conceived accidentally or immediately on cessation of use of Depo-Provera has also not been studied.

Problems such as amenorrhoea (absence of menstruation), irregular bleeding, generalised weakness, migraine headaches and severe abdominal cramps have been considered by the researchers to be "non-serious". From a woman user perspective, these side-effects could hamper daily activities and significantly affect well-being. We must remember that contraceptives are targeted at women in the prime of their lives, and such debilitating side-effects cannot be side-lined as "non-serious".

Equally worrisome is the opinion of the manufacturer's that side-effects like irregular bleeding can be "dealt" with by counselling alone. Besides the serious implications of blood-loss in an already anaemic population, experts have pointed out that menstrual cycle patterns may be a fundamental determinant of women's health status and that alterations in menstrual function may influence many disease processes including the natural resistance to metastatic spread of cancer. Similarly, prolonged amenorrhoea in the absence of pregnancy is not a 'harmless', but a serious medical event causing endometrial atrophy, which could have a bearing on the woman's future fertility status (Sathyamala, 2000).

The PMS study on Depo-Provera also flouts international guidelines for ethical medical research. The use of lactating women as study subjects is a violation of the Code of the Council for International Organisations of Medical Sciences (CIOMS). Further, the administration of Depo-Provera during lactation could have a serious adverse effect on the health of breast-feeding women because of the association with demineralisation of the bones.

Despite its problematic entry on the Indian scene, Depo-Provera is now available in the market, easily procured over the counter. A recent study by Sama, a Delhi-based health group, revealed that Depo-Provera was also being prescribed in government hospitals in Delhi. Lack of informed consent and side-effects of the drug were points repeatedly raised by the women interviewed. The study revealed that 42 out of 50 women were not given any information about the side effects, and 48 out of 52 women reported problems after using the injectable and each woman had multiple problems (Sama, 2002). With such a situation in a public hospital, the state of affairs in private establishments can be well imagined.

While the Depo-saga relates to spacing methods of contraception, another well known case of private bodies carrying out research and contraceptive outreach is that of quinacrine—a permanent method of sterilisation.

**The Quinacrine Story**

Around 1996-97, it came to light that doctors, unregistered medical practitioners and NGOs in West Bengal, Karnataka, Uttar Pradesh, Gujarat, Delhi and Chandigarh for more than 20 years had been using quinacrine, an anti-malarial drug, to sterilise poor and illiterate slum and rural women. Quinacrine is a sclerosing agent, which burns the uterine tissues causing inflammation and the formation of scabs in the uterine lining. The scar tissues block the inner end of the fallopian tubes and prevent the sperm from reaching the ovum.

The short term side effects of quinacrine sterilisation (QS) are severe abdominal pain and cramps, fever, yellow pungent smelling discharge, lower back pain, nausea, headaches and itching. More disturbing are its long-term risks. Quinacrine is a known mutagen and past laboratory studies have pointed to potential risks of cancer, birth defects and toxicity. Moreover, some women become pregnant despite undergoing QS; because the method is imprecise since one cannot control the direction in which quinacrine pellets are inserted into the uterus and know precisely how they will dissolve in the uterus and form scabs to block the fallopian tubes. The possibility of women dropping out of the treatment after the first insertion may leave the blockage of the fallopian tube incomplete. This could lead to the danger of ectopic pregnancy, which in Indian conditions where the health infrastructure is poor and women have little access to health services, can prove to be fatal. Also unknown is the effect of QS on pregnant women and the foetus, since women in early pregnancy may unknowingly seek QS.

Developed in the early 70s by Chilean scientist Jaime Zipper, QS has been actively promoted by Dr. Elton Kessel of the International Federation of Family Health (IFFH) and Dr. Stephen Mumford of the Centre for Research on Population and Security (CRPS), both based in the US. Elton Kessel and Mumford first collaborated on Quinacrine trials through the International Fertility Research Programme (IFRP), Research Triangle Park, North Carolina, USA, an institution of which Kessel was the founder member. The IFRP has subsequently been renamed the Family Health International (FHI), which describes itself as a non-profit US based organisation dedicated to contraceptive development, family planning and reproductive health and AIDS prevention around the world. Through the FHI, Kessel and his colleagues made two attempts to get the approval of the USFDA on Quinacrine sterilisations, but failed. Currently, Kessel is Secretary General of IFFH, while Dr. J.K. Jain, ex-BJP MP and owner of the Jain Medical Centre in New Delhi, is its President.

Kessel, Mumford and their colleagues literally traverse the globe with Quinacrine pellets in their suitcases, urging gynaecologists at meetings and conferences to try Quinacrine sterilisation. For instance, Kessel turned up at a meeting of the Patiala Obstetrics and Gynaecological Society in January, 1997 and delivered an oration entitled, '100,000 Quinacrine Sterilisations'. "Probably the most important need", he claimed, "is to encourage expansion of Quinacrine sterilisation in the private sector as an 'off-label drug' as it is approved almost everywhere for treatment of malaria. Dr. Maya Sood, HOD, Gyn. and Obs., Lady Hardinge Medical College, New Delhi, revealed in the documentary film, The Yellow Haze, that she was going to meet Kessel shortly in Agra. Similarly, Dr. Sneh Vishwanathan, Consultant, Parivar Seva Sansthan (Marie Stopes, India) also reported having met Kessel in a conference in Karachi in 1994, and becoming convinced about the Quinacrine sterilisation method."

The ubiquitous CRPS was also present at the Global Forum at the Fourth World Conference on Women, Beijing (September, 1995) where they promoted Quinacrine as a way to improve women's health and reduce maternal mortality. In a classic example of doublespeak, their training video was produced by the "Empowerment Project". Fortunately, a number of women's health activists were at hand to challenge them.

Sarah G. Epstein, another vehement advocate of Quinacrine, along with her husband Donald A. Collins, also a population consultant, attended the Beijing Conference to carry out pro-Quinacrine propaganda. For two weeks prior to the Conference, they toured Chinese villages and cities with a group from the Population Institute, Washington DC. They met local health service officials to promote Quinacrine as an effective, safe and inexpensive sterilisation method. Epstein and Collins, not incidentally, are also on the Board of the Federation for American Immigration Reform (FAIR).

Through these ardent advocates of QS, the method spread to remote corners of the developing world. In West Bengal alone, according to conservative estimates, more than 30,000 women have undergone QS since the late 70s. In the mid-1990s, the Contraceptive and Health Innovations Project (CHIP Trust) in Bangalore was involved in a two year project to sterilise 25,000 women by the method. A government hospital, Lady Hardinge Medical College through its rural outreach centre on the outskirts of Delhi was carrying out clinical trials on women who were unaware of the risks or that they were part of a trial. Actual figures of QS are hard to determine because the practice is unregulated and the doctors promoting the method are mainly private doctors and unregistered rural practitioners.

It is significant that for all these years, QS was not an

approved method in the country. It did not have the approval of any national drug agency like the DGCI whose permission is essential for the trial or use of any new drug/method in the country. Nor is QS approved by international agencies like the WHO or Food and Drug Administration (FDA has, however, recently allowed limited human trials in the USA). In fact, although the proponents and distributors of the method like Dr. Jain claimed that they were conducting 'clinical trials' of the method, no approval was ever sought for the same, nor have the results been made public, beyond loose claims of its alleged safety (Saheli, 1997).

Following an intense campaign by women's groups in several parts of the country, the DGCI in December, 1997 banned the use of quinacrine for female sterilisation. To add weight to the prohibition, the Supreme Court, on 16th March, 1998, in response to a petition filed by AIDWA and faculty of the Centre for Social Medicine and Community Health, JNU, passed an order upholding the ban on QS. While the Court did uphold the ban, and directed a official gazette notification, it refused to direct the prosecution of the guilty with retrospective effect. It is only future violations which are punishable. Implementation of the ban has been left to the State Governments.

In India, despite the ban, the use of QS has been reported in some pockets of West Bengal (no information on other parts of the country). The practice has only gone 'underground' and the price for QS gone up. Quinacrine pellets for QS are still being distributed among others by one of its staunchest advocates in Calcutta, Dr. Biral Mullick. From his centre in Kolkata, he also mails to doctors in India QS Newsletters published in the US by the global promoters of QS. Recently, the Calcutta-based National Association for Reproductive and Child Health of India (NARCHI) petitioned the DGCI to rescind the ban. To persuade the DGCI decision, NARCHI sent with the appeal news clips of QS trials in countries like the USA, Chile and China (Dasgupta, R., 2000).

## Ethics of Industry-Sponsored Research

The shift from 'neutral' bodies conducting research to research by bodies that have a stake in the outcome of the research has deep implications. Post Marketing Surveillance by pharmaceutical companies in lieu of Phase IV clinical trials conducted by impartial scientific bodies is another outcome of the liberalised economy. These trends are directly related to the phenomenon of the market, where profit is the king. It must not be forgotten that India is one of the largest markets for contraceptives in the world. With almost 40 million potential users the Indian contraceptive market is larger than the entire population of Switzerland, Norway, Sweden, and Australia put together. Little wonder that multinational pharmaceutical companies have been consistently wooing this market with aggressive propaganda.

Industry-sponsored research has given rise to a gamut of issues which need to be addressed on a priority basis. When "efficiency-based" standards, and supremacy of "local standards", which are lower than international standards prevail, there is cause for serious alarm (as in HIV drug trials in Africa). Many investigators have argued for dual standards. They claim that there should be different ethical standards for developing and developed countries (Lancet, 1998, quoted by Singh *et al.*, 2000). There is considerable opposition to this from the scientific community as well; for example inclusion of placebo groups in testing of a variety of treatment regimens with AZT for prevention of HIV transmission to infants by women with AIDS in Africa has been challenged (Lurie and Wolfe, 1997, quoted by Singh *et al.*, 2000). The marketeers of Depo Provera and the proponents of QS have also made similar arguments and argued that the actual living conditions in the country and issues like high maternal mortality should be taken into account when considering ethical guidelines, and Western standards of safety and risks should not be applied. (Singh *et al.*, 2000).

At the international level, moves to amend standard international ethical codes are a cause for serious concern for all those engaged in matters of medical ethics and their implications for the health of people. The pressures to modify the Helsinki Declaration in the recent past were in part an effort to make clinical research easier in developing countries. The first change sought was to permit "proxy consent" that would eliminate the need for individual informed consent by obtaining permission from a governmental or non-governmental body in a position of authority. The second change sought to stipulate that the standard of care to be provided to people enrolled in clinical trials need not be 'the best-proven care' but rather 'best care available in the country'.

The implications of such moves are directly seen in the watering down of the provisions for mandatory informed consent in the 'Ethical Guidelines on Biomedical Research Involving Human Subjects' released by the Indian Council of Medical Research (ICMR) or the 'ICMR Code', 2000. Following this prescription, the ICMR Code, in its section on "International Collaboration/Assistance in Bio-Medical/Health research" does not provide adequate safeguards against exploitation of research subjects from a developing country. For instance, by talking about "best possible nationally available care", the Code allows for by-passing international standards, which will work against research subjects.

**The ICMR Code: A Critique and Some Recommendations**

Ethical violations in contraceptive trials and epidemiological research by scientific bodies which set standards for the whole country, such as the ICMR demonstrate the need for public debate and intervention.

In 1997, Draft guidelines were issued by the ICMR seeking input from health professionals and activists. The 'Consultative Document on Ethical Guidelines on Biomedical Research Involving Human Subjects' was drafted by the Central Ethics Committee on Human research (CECHR) under the chairmanship of Justice M.N. Venkatachaliah, who at the time was also chairman of the National Human Rights Commission (NHRC).

Regional public debates were held in Calcutta, Mumbai, Hyderabad and New Delhi. Women's and health groups at the forefront of campaigns highlighting violations in medical ethics were not invited to most of these meetings. Saheli had submitted a detailed critique and list of recommendations. After four years, the final document, christened the ICMR Code, was released in September, 2000.

The Code includes many areas not covered by the sketchy 1980 ICMR Policy Statement on Ethical Considerations Involved in Research on Human Subjects, *e.g.* human genetics research, organ transplantation, epidemiological research and Assisted Reproductive Technologies. Widening the scope of the document is an encouraging sign of the attempt to keep pace with the challenges posed by scientific and technological developments.

However, the Code fails to acknowledge changing social trends, especially in the context of gender and class inequalities in Indian society. There are detailed recommendations about "Ethical Review Procedures" and the setting up of Institutional Ethical Committees. Yet, these details appear to be bureaucratic procedural matters, and do not embody the spirit of ensuring ethical bio-medical research. Ethical guidelines should go beyond technicalities and build effective safeguards so that the unequal power relationship between researchers and subjects is neutralised and no new avenues of exploitation of research subjects are opened up. It is crucial that the basic principles be stated clearly and unambiguously. The current document falls short of these objectives.

Contentious issues remain relating to newer technologies like genetic research, organ transplantation etc., which need to be publicly debated with groups working in these areas. As a women's organisation, we shall here address the shortcomings in the Code in areas in which we have been directly engaged.

**Informed Consent**

Informed Consent is central to ethical biomedical research, but has not received adequate attention. The Draft undermines the cardinal principle of informed consent in the interest of "the overall purpose and importance of research." The possibility of "waiver of informed consent" is unacceptable, since 'emergency' is left undefined. A new section headed "Obligations of the investigators regarding informed consent" highlights important issues such as deception, undue influence and intimidation while giving consent; evidence of informed consent; renewal of informed consent during an on-going trial etc. However, some issues which still need consideration are:

(*i*) Information about potential risks and benefits should be provided verbally and in writing in English/Hindi, and in vernacular whenever necessary.

(*ii*) A social worker (not the doctor alone) should be involved in counselling. During written informed consent, the signature should be witnessed by a person not related with the trial.

(*iii*) For research involving the whole community/large group, the consent of the village elder and/or community leader should not be considered adequate. Proxy consent should not be permitted.

(*iv*) Where a new study proposes to use samples collected for a previous study, consent given for the earlier study cannot be deemed to apply to the new study.

(*v*) Even when the research design involves minimal risk (*e.g.* only collecting data from subjects' records) the Ethical Committee should make a case-by-case judgement about waiving informed consent.

(*vi*) Researchers should not be allowed to disclose the identity of the participants to those not associated with the trial, without seeking permission from the Ethical Committee.

(*vii*) Health insurance should be mandatory for trial participants, provision for which should be communicated while obtaining informed consent.

**Assisted Reproductive Technlogies (ARTs)**

The ICMR (Draft Document) has been recently thrown open for public debate. This is an area in which no previous ethical guidelines exist in India. Yet, the draft document, rather than highlight the ethical, moral and legal dilemmas likely to be encountered at an individual, familial and social level, outlines the procedural aspects of Assisted Reproduction in great detail.

The Guidelines reveal biases which could work against the interests of certain sections who are not within the narrowly defined confines of the family, *e.g.* single parents, non-heterosexuals etc. The notion of "legitimacy" of children needs to be re-defined keeping in minds the custodial rights of mothers.

Ethical guidelines should not accept social stigma attached to infertility as a norm. Societies have evolved social ways for childless couples to deal with infertility, for instance, adoption, foster-parenthood, etc.

The Code reinforces conservative attitudes by recommending matching of religious and ethnic background for donor insemination. Even the new draft guidelines for ART put up for discussion by ICMR continue to harbour the prejudice of finding the religion and ethnic background of the donor. Issues like religion and educational level have no bearing on genetic inheritance and should not be considerations during donor selection.

Moreover, the Code has not been drafted keeping in mind a long-term perspective. Scope should be left in the guidelines to consider introduction of new technologies and the debates ensuing from their potential use.

**Contraceptive Research**

Lack of separate attention to this area of research in the Draft was a serious lacuna pointed out by us. The Code now carries a paragraph on contraceptives under the general heading of "Special Concerns". This paragraph does, however, highlight three crucial issues—informed consent and information about the alternatives available, proper follow-up—even when a subject has withdrawn from the trial—as in Norplant, and follow-up of children born due to contraceptive failure.

Yet, we feel that the issue of contraceptive research deserves more attention. The bulk of contraceptive research is targeted towards women, a section of society that has lower nutritional levels, poor access to health facilities and a lack of decision making power over sexuality. Secondly, most of the emerging contraceptive technologies have multi-system effects, and require more careful studies in order to ensure their long-term safety *vis-à-vis* women's health and their future progeny.

All aspects of contraceptive research must respect the diverse knowledge and needs of women, as defined by women. Further, fertility and pregnancy are not diseases, but a normal part of a woman's life and must be understood as such. Since contraceptives are used by healthy women and men in the prime of their lives, the risks-benefit evaluation has to be different from that used on drugs/procedures for treatment of diseases.

Hence, we suggest the following broad guidelines (inspired by the Canadian Women's Committee on Population and Development: Bill of Rights for Contraceptive Research, Development and Use, 1993) within which contraceptive research must be conducted:

**Contraceptive Research and Development**

1. Hazardous contraceptives, and contraceptives with potential for abuse should not be promoted. Instead, such methods should be promoted which:

    - enhance women's health and well-being;
    - are user-controlled;
    - are reversible in the case of spacing methods;
    - meet women's needs at various points in their life cycle;
    - exhibit demonstrable advantages over existing contraceptives.

2. Research must assess the degree of risk to children conceived as a result of contraceptive failure.
3. More resources must be allocated to the development of safer methods of contraception, such as barrier methods, that offer protection from sexually transmitted diseases, especially HIV; and also to the development of male contraceptives.

4. As part of formal research processes, mechanisms must be introduced which facilitate equal participation of women's health activists and potential contraceptive users in decision-making and advisory bodies involved in:

   - setting research priorities;
   - monitoring on-going research;
   - defining the criteria for safety;
   - reviewing research findings and assessing the acceptability of a method to proceed from one research stage to another.

5. Contraceptive research must be subject to review by multidisciplinary ethics committees.
6. There should be transparency in contraceptive research, including: criteria for determining research priorities, information on research protocols, process and findings; criteria for determining safety; funding and patent information.

**Contraceptive Testing, Evaluation, Approval and Monitoring**

1. Written informed consent must be obtained from all the participants of research trials in accordance with the guidelines laid down in Informed Consent.
2. Researchers, government and funding institutions are responsible for ensuring the safety of trial participants, and liable in case of damage to health/life of the trial participants or their future progeny.
3. Participants must be informed of their right to withdraw from trials at any time. Voluntary withdrawals must get due weightage during trial evaluations.
4. To determine whether a contraceptive is appropriate for a particular country, trials must take place within that country. Participants in these trials must reflect the make-up of women who will be using the contraceptives.

5. Long-term monitoring and follow-up of trial participants and children born to them during or after trials must be undertaken to determine the effects of the contraceptive technologies over time.
6. Contraceptive trials should immediately cease if the potential arises for serious risk to trial participants.
7. Users' responses to and assessment of the contraceptive method under review must be recognised as valid research findings and incorporated into the evaluation process.
8. Independent mechanisms must be established to monitor research trials to ensure compliance with international ethical standards.

**Post-Marketing Surveillance**

While equating Post-Marketing Surveillance (PMS) to the Phase IV clinical trial, the Code disclaims responsibility to oversee its results, by claiming that this is "outside the purview of the ethical committee". The Code does, however, highlight one area of frequent violation of ethics. "A physician investigator ...should ensure that patients understand and remember that the drug is experimental and that its benefits for the condition under study are yet unproven." In drugs like Depo-Provera, which are easily available even over-the-counter, this precaution has not been followed, thus making a farce of the PMS. There is an urgent need to provide stringent guidelines to govern PMS.

Our experience with PMS of contraceptives demonstrates the problems inherent in the concept. PMS being conducted by the pharmaceutical company which stands to gain directly, defies scientific objectivity.

Some recommendations to monitor PMS are :

(*i*) Monitoring mechanisms should be an integral part of the licensing agreement.

(*ii*) PMS should be carried out within a defined period after approval for mareting is given.

(*iii*) Information should be provided on the package of the drug/device clearly stating that it is undergoing PMS.

(*iv*) Adequate information must include all known potential side-effects, however rare.

(*v*) Treatment plan for side effects/complications must be part of the ethical clearance prior to commencement of marketing/PMS.

(*vi*) Mechanisms to award damages in case of complications, serious side-effects, long-term problems, etc. must be set into motion.

(*vii*) License/Registration should be provisional until results of PMS are available.

(*viii*) Results of PMS should be subject to independent expert analysis.

**Newer Developments**

Some new developments have disturbing implications. Most developing countries have poor regulatory processes to conduct even Phase I and Phase II trials, hence it is cheaper and simpler for interested parties to conduct these trials in developing countries provided the data were acceptable to regulatory agencies in the US or in Europe. India is poised for a major expansion in the clinical trial business for several reasons. First, it has a well-developed infrastructure. Second, it has highly trained personnel and speciality equipment available at a fraction of what it would cost in a developed country. Third, it has a large population base so that trial subjects can be recruited readily. Finally, it has a relatively lax regulatory process and a government that has committed to implement product patents by the year 2005 under the WTO rules. All these factors make it very attractive for pharmaceutical companies and Clinical Research Organisations (CROs) to conduct trials in India (D'Mello, 2000).

For instance, according to *The Economist*, "India promises to become a world centre for testing new medicines" (January 29, 2000, quoted in D'Mello, 2000). CROs which undertake clinical trials and other services for pharmaceutical companies are beginning to find a location advantage in India. Quintiles, a large CRO based in North Carolina and Covance, a CRO based in New Jersey, have started conducting clinical trials in India and are expanding their operations. Corporations like Nicholas Piramal have begun a new clinical trials business, and Max India has entered into a deal with the Harvard Medical School to conduct clinical trials in India and other underdeveloped countries. According to the same news report, a Covance vice-president (global safety and medical therapeutics) expected "tremendous" return on investing in India's infrastructure for conducting clinical trials.

It is claimed that a large part of the total expenditure of around $500 million that is required to discover and develop a drug is spent on clinical trials. Phase III trials use a number of human subjects. If clinical testing can be done faster and cheaper, the additional returns from an earlier launch may fetch "millions of dollars of extra revenue to the patent's owners". Clinical trials in India can be cheaper and faster. Moreover, India's billion potential guinea-pigs suffer not just from tropical diseases such as malaria and tuberculosis, but increasingly from ailments such as cancer, heart disease and AIDS, which trouble rich countries. The Head of Quintile's India venture, Ferzaan Engineer says that for some diseases research in India can dramatically reduce the time for commercial launch of new therapies.

The shifting of research by for-profit organisations to the Third World must be viewed in the light of these norms—both national and international—of medical research. The ICMR Code merely skims over this issue. "Academic institutions conducting research in alliance with industries/commercial companies require a strong review to probe possible conflicts of interest between scientific responsibilities of researchers and business interests (*e.g.* ownership or part-ownership of a company developing a new product). While the Code leaves it to institutions to set in motion "self-regulatory processes to monitor, prevent and resolve such conflicts of interests", it does recommend that prospective participants in research "should also be informed of the sponsorship of the research, so that they can be aware of the potential for conflicts of interest and commercial aspects of the research."

But in an increasingly corporatised world, such vague guidelines on conflict of interest as stated in the ICMR Code are unlikely to reign in the unethical and irresponsible trends like we have seen as in the cases of Depo-Provera, QS and AZT etc. In fact, before we end, we need to at least outline the plethora of concerns that this unleashes for us.

## Corporate Conduct : Accountability is the First Victim

On one hand, health groups have been working for greater safeguards for peoples' health in the context of medical research and clinical trials. But failing such protection, the next natural question is the issue of what recourse a trial subject has for adequate medical attention or compensation for damages during the entire process.

Unlike the pre-liberalised scenario where the state could be held responsible for the nature, conduct, results and follow-up of clinical trials on human subjects through its health programmes, we have now entered an era of increased vulnerability of peoples' health. From being a 'trial subject', today a woman buying Depo-Provera over the counter or undergoing QS in a private clinic has been turned into a 'consumer' with little recourse for justice in a land where the consumer protection movement is yet to find a footing, the inclusion of medical services under the Consumer Protection Act notwithstanding.

Add to this the issue of accountability in the context of corporate takeovers and the scenario becomes cause for greater concern. As we all know, when Dow Chemical took over Union Carbide Corporation (UCC) in February, 2001, it created the largest chemical corporation in the world. With the merger, Dow took on UCC's assets, but has refused to take on its liabilities—the fallout of the world's worst industrial disaster in Bhopal caused by faulty plant design and gross negligence, which according to survivors' organisations killed more than 2,000 people in the immediate aftermath, and about ten times that number over the following 18 years.

Yet, the Indian Government attempted (unsuccessfully) to dilute the original charges of culpable homicide against prime accused Warren Anderson—Chairman of Union Carbide at the time of the disaster. This development illustrates the concern of the Indian Government that prosecuting Warren Anderson, the head of a transnational corporation would "jeopardise the investment climate". Only sustained pressure from people's organisations has forced the Madhya Pradesh Government to announce that it will approach the Supreme Court in a bid to hold Dow Chemicals accountable (Indian Express, October 20, 2002).

Such corporate takeovers and business alliances, though seemingly far removed from people's lives, have a far-reaching impact. In 1995, a merger of Sweden's Pharmacia with Upjohn of the US resulted in Pharmacia and Upjohn. One can only wonder what impact the Pfizer take-over of Pharmacia-Upjohn, the manufacturers of Depo-Provera, in a stock-for-stock transaction valued at $60 billion, will have on women users of Depo-Provera in India. The merger, announced in July, 2002 is described as creating "a strategic opportunity that immediately creates a global pharmaceutical company with unsurpassed resources and capabilities".

Such developments give rise to a plethora of questions. How can industrial giants be made to shoulder the liabilities of companies taken over? What are the resources that affected women can garner to fight pharmaceutical giants like these? And what on the other hand, are the strategies with which women can be enabled to safeguard themselves against NGOs, CROs and other private institutions that also dominate the field?

**End Note**

Conclusions are not possible in a paper like the present one.

But a reiteration of some of the questions raised might help us to find answers. While enunciating good guidelines for ethical conduct of clinical research are essential, they are clearly not enough. The problem is more fundamental. Who will ensure that the priorities of research go beyond generating profit to address issues of public health and safety? Who will ensure that trials are conducted within the ethical guidelines? By what means will unethical investigators be held accountable? Finally, if there is no political will or if national agencies do not have the political clout how can we ensure that they will be able to enforce the guidelines?

New ethical guidelines, in addition to keeping pace with scientific developments, must prioritise safeguarding the rights, health and well-being of research subjects. Corporate profits cannot be put ahead of individual well-being. The manner in which political ideology permeates medical research makes it imperative to develop a pro-people, pro-woman definition of "overall purpose" of research.

## REFERENCES


Brennan, T.A. (1999): 'Proposed Revisions to the Declaration of Helsinki - Will they Weaken the Ethical Principles Underlying Human Research?' *New England Journal of Medicine:* Vol. 341, No. 7.

Canadian Women's Committee on Population and Development (1993): Bill of Rights for Contraceptive Research, Development and Use.

Dasgupta, R. (2000): 'Status of Quinacrine Sterilisation in India: A Report' paper presented at the Workshop on 'Bioethics of Quinacrine Sterilisation, Informed Consent and Contraceptive Trials: Implications for Human Rights of Women,' Kolkata, December (Unpublished).

D'Mello B., September (2000): 'Transnational Pharmaceutical Corporations and Neo-Liberal Ethics in Business in India', Unpublished.

Hartosh Singh Bal (2002): 'MP wants Dow to clean up Carbide Mess,' Indian Express, October 20.

Indian Council of Medical Research, (2000): 'Ethical Guidelines for Biomedical Research on Human Subjects', ICMR, September.

Saheli (1997): 'Quinacrine: The Sordid Story of Chemical Sterilisation of Women—A Saheli Report', New Delhi.

Sama, (September 2002): 'A Study on Women's Experiences with Depo Provera: A Preliminary Report,' New Delhi.

Sathyamala, C. (2001): 'An Epidemiological Review of the Injectable Contraceptive, Depo-Provera', Medico Friend Circle and Forum for Women's Health.

Singh, N. and Shree Mulay (2000): 'A Critique of Ethical Guidelines for Clinical Research from the Perspective of Women's Rights and Social Justice', paper presented at the Workshop on 'Bioethics of Quinacrine Sterilisation, Informed Consent and Contraceptive Trials: Implications for Human Rights of Women,' Kolkata, December (Unpublished).

United Nations Population Fund, 'Programme Review and Strategy Development: India' (Undated).

www.pfizer.com.

# NEGLECTED TODAY : FORGOTTEN TOMORROW

# 14

# THE RIGHT TO GROW

## An Unaffordable Luxury

***Children's Rights in Goa (CRG)***

*The poor man dies because he cannot afford to live.*

—Dr. Norman Bethune

In India the growth of 52 per cent of children under five is stunted. The causes of stunted growth are attributed to low weight at birth (because of the poor health of the mothers), inadequate feeding and repeated illnesses (Bellamy, 2000). Goa prides itself on its relatively better conditions of health and literacy and a higher standard of living than other parts of the country.

In this paper, our intention is to explore a face of Goa that remains invisible in all discourses and representations of Goa. A Goa in which, literacy levels are low, proper sanitation and hygiene are inaccessible luxuries, and the right to grow is literally and metaphorically speaking, denied to its children. This is a Goa that is inhabited by families who have come from other states, in search of a livelihood because of acute poverty in the states of their origin.

We would like to argue that this is an integral part of Goa and requires recognition. The people inhabiting this Goa have played an invaluable role in contributing to the development of Goa. However, their own development and their right to growth has been compromised. To illustrate this let us look at the health of children of families residing in Sanvordem-Curchorem, involved in the unloading and loading of mining ore.

Some of the children in this region attend an open school run by Children's Rights in Goa (CRG) in a classroom of the Chandrabhaga Technical Institute. We have had the opportunity of working with children in this area for three years. They live in Chamomal village Curchorem which has the stacking yard where the iron, bauxite and manganese ores from the mines around the area are brought in trucks and sent out of Goa by wagons. Our observations are based on our interaction with children and their families as well as the local primary health centre. CRG has also done a formal survey of 20 families in the region in March, 2002.

**Nature of Households and Living Conditions**

Many of the households have lived in Goa for over 5 years. One family has been living here for the past 21 years, but they are viewed as outsiders with no right to ration cards, water connections, permanent housing or the right to be accepted as members of Goan society.

They hail from Hubli, Gadag, Bijapur and various parts of Karnataka. Most visit their home state in June, once the monsoon starts in Goa and return around September. Those who work as agricultural labourers during this time reported that they earn Rs. 20 per day. They are driven to come to Goa because they are unable to make a living in their home state. Many who work here support parents or children who continue to stay in their villages.

The households surveyed were mostly found to be comprised of nuclear families. Ten families comprised more than six members and 4 families had more than eight members. Only in a few instances were any of the grandparents staying as members of the household. There were a total of 51 children living in Goa amongst these families. In numerous cases some of the siblings stay in their villages with a parent or relatives.

There was one case of one family in which the man and his six-year-old son live in Goa while the woman remains in the village with their two daughters. The father works most of the day, coming home at lunch time to give his son his food, and dropping him off to the CRG school after this. Much of the time this child depends on his neighbours for social contact and sustenance.

In another case Salma stays in Goa with her two sons and a daughter. The father stays in Hubli with one son and his mother. Interestingly, he works as a truck driver and sends Salma Rs. 1000 per month. Salma earns around Rs. 200 per week, loading and unloading wagons.

In numerous cases both the parents work. Take the case of six-year-old Mahesh who is left in the care of his older sister, as both the parents work. As she goes to school, he is alone at home for parts of the day.

A number of the children who come to the CRG open school bring along their younger siblings who have been entrusted to their care.

The contractor provides them housing, hence those who work on the wagons do not pay any rent. The houses are temporary structures made mainly of tin sheets with one or two small rooms. Some have cement floors but others have just mud and there is hardly any ventilation. Most cook and sleep in the same room which makes it more congested. They have light connections but water is scarce. There are no toilet facilities so they have to go out in the open.

**Conditions of Work**

Out of 20 families, 14 couples worked at wagon loading and unloading and the others are involved in varied occupations working as painters, mechanics and domestic labourers. For wagon loading and unloading there are no real fixed hours of work. They are employed by a contractor. Whenever the wagons come they were asked to do the job, even at times through the night. If there are no wagons they are given an off. They are able to unload at least two wagons per head which, earns them approximately Rs. 80 per wagon. Both husband and wife do the work of unloading and some times older children help them and the family is paid a round sum of Rs. 100. Children are paid Rs. 20 to 40 for their labour.

## Child Labour

We found one instance of child labour for every two households surveyed. Out of ten child labourers eight were 10 years and below.

Small children often accompany their parents to the work-site and are exposed to dust pollution. As they become older they begin to help their parents with the loading and unloading operations. From the households surveyed, five children, two boys and three girls in the age group from 9 to 12 years were found to be engaged in the loading and unloading operations, earning between Rs. 20 to Rs. 40 per day. Children were also found to be involved in other occupations.

Nine-year-old Rizu works in a bar and earns Rs. 550 per month. 14-year-old Keshav works in a garage and earns Rs. 500 per month and earns more than his father who earns Rs. 300 per month working as a *hamali*. Two boys earn Rs. 20 per day collecting plastic. One boy earns Rs. 20 per day selling lottery tickets.

## Educational Status

When we talk about educational status of these families, out of 20 families, among the adults only nine say they have been to school for basic education. Interestingly, five out of the nine are women, one of whom studied up to 10th std.

Out of 51 children only 16 attend formal school *i.e.* government and aided schools. 15 attend the non-formal school run by Children's Rights in Goa .

## Nature of Health Problems

Dust pollution is the most dangerous and widespread fall out of ore transportation. Due to intense pollution of dust around and in the mining areas, their work of loading and unloading the wagons most of them suffer various respiratory problems such as tuberculosis and asthma. According to the report given by the Health Centre every month there are 10 to 12 tuberculosis cases.

According to a study done by the Sanvordem Citizens Forum, a body that has been actively demanding the shifting of these operations to a less habited area, and has even filed a case in the High Court in this matter, every resident of Sanvordem has been afflicted with an illness related to dust pollution and has spent money for their treatment (Naik no date).

Ten-year-old Laxmi and her younger brother are suffering from ear problems which her family said was related to the loading activities. According to a study on the impact of the mining industry:

> *"Sound pollution specially during the nights by heavy earth moving machinery causes impaired hearing, mental problems and disturbance in sleeping for the population neighbouring loading points."(ibid.)*

Lack of sanitation and running water result in other illnesses such as diarrhoea and worm infestation.

Another problem that has serious ramifications for the health of the young girl and her offspring is the issue of early marriages. In the course of interaction with children in the open school, we have found young girls getting married at the age of 15 to 16 years. Parents often see this as affording protection to their daughters who they are otherwise unable to supervise or protect.

Most of the adults interviewed said they preferred going to private doctors. One woman stated that a neighbour had taken her child who had burn injuries to a government hospital. She insisted that the child died and when his body was brought back home by the parents the eyes, heart and kidney had been removed. It was difficult to ascertain what exactly had happened in this case as this family went back to their village shortly after the death of this child. But the woman interviewee vowed she would never go to a government hospital. This was a view that was shared by others but with lesser intensity.

A common reason given by adults for going to the doctor was body ache and/or headache for which they were treated by private doctors with various tonics and tablets.

Unfortunately there are no health check-ups conducted by the contractor at all, nor does the contractor reimburse any medical expenses incurred by them. The workers have to come for treatment on their own. As no proper record is maintained, it is difficult to ascertain what treatment they have received and whether the treatment has been completed or not.

## Some Issues

Article 24 of the Convention of the Rights of the Child states that children and young people under 18 years have the right to the enjoyment of the highest attainable standard of health and it is the duty of the State to ensure this right to each and every child without any discrimination. Child health care is not only the provision of medical care . It means the provision of comprehensive health care from the time of conception till the child becomes an independent adult. This means ensuring that :

- the pregnant mother is looked after so that her baby will be healthy
- each infant is cared for by trained adults in the absence of their parents enabling children to go to school instead of looking after their younger siblings.
- that contractors be made responsible for providing decent living conditions to the people they employ for loading/unloading operations.
- that the primary health centre play an active role in monitoring the health of the residents of this area.
- that the government be proactive in reducing the hazard of pollution and ensuring more humane conditions of work and living in this area.

## REFERENCES

Bellamy, Carol 2000: in UNICEF, *The Progress of Nation 2000,* UNICEF, New York:15.

Naik, Niraj (no date): 'Everything you want to know about Goa's Mining Industry' *Impact of Mining : A Case Study* (available with CRG, Goa).

15

# GENDER, AGEING AND HEALTH IN GOA

*Fatima da Silva Gracias*

The International Year of the Older Person (1999) and the World Assembly on Ageing held at Spain in April, 2002, brought into focus issues concerning the elderly in many parts of the world. Until recently the subject of ageing was not much discussed in India. The older population in India has steadily increased in the last few decades as a result of decline in fertility, mortality and other factors. Therefore, issues concerning the elderly need attention and are likely to be one of the major concerns in the near future. This paper is going to review the position of ageing women in Goa and their health conditions.

The report on 'Ageing in Goa at the Turn of the Third Millennium' published this year (2002) by the Research Institute for Women, Goa, does not provide a rosy picture about the situation of the ageing population in Goa (RIW, 2002). The report has classified the older persons into two brackets 'the third age' (65 to 75) and 'the fourth age' (75 and the above).

In Goa, among the ageing population a large number are women. The feminisation of ageing is becoming more pronounced with women living longer then men for reasons mentioned elsewhere in this paper. The gender difference is evident in the "fourth age" group, with women outnumbering men. Among the ageing population over 60 per cent are women. Elderly women can be divided in two groups those who are active and those who are dependent on others for care.

Ageing is a part of a person's life span. Today, ageing in Goa for both men and women is a difficult process. In the last 40 years Goa has gone through a whole lot of changes—a period of transition following the transfer of power from that a colony of Portugal to being part of Indian Union. This brought about changes in the scenario namely urbanisation, changes from agricultural economy, decline in the institution of joint family, paucity of adequate housing in growing towns and out migration (Gracias, 2000). Migration too has brought with it problems, some of which have affected the older group.

The elderly in Goa no longer enjoy the same status in the family and in the society as they did in the past. Various pressures of life, growth of nuclear family and lack of space in urban areas are steadily detaching the younger generation from the elder members of their family. In modern society only the young and resourceful are considered useful. Those who do not produce are becoming less important and many times are considered a liability (Desai, 1999).

In this state, the family is the traditional social institution for the care of the elderly women. The family is the principal source of support and security in old age. A majority of women in the third and fourth age group live with their families. That is with their spouse or one of their married adult sons or daughters, unmarried children or extended families (RIW, 2002). In the third and fourth age groups besides married women and widows, there are also unmarried ones mainly in the Christian community.

The position of the elder women depends on socio-economic conditions of the family. A few have independent means of support. Majority of them face problems of poor economic means and age related ailments. They have no independent means of support. A sizeable number of widows and unmarried women are dependent on their families for support and care.

Among the lower classes, many women continue working far beyond their working age as unskilled labourers, domestic servants or as vendors. They have problems supporting themselves with meagre incomes. The question of support and care for the elderly women requires to be dealt with. There is need to make them self-sufficient so that they need not be a burden to their families.

While the family provides care and support, the older women in turn often contribute to the well-being of the family in terms of their support in childcare, caring of another elderly family members, etc. Older women take care of their old spouses, older parents or siblings in the fourth age group sometimes in their late 80s or 90s. Very often infants and small children are left with the grandmothers or an unmarried grand aunt while the parents are at work. At other times, mothers and aunts are asked by the migrant children to look after their homes. And of late many grandmothers have travelled overseas for a period of time to help in the care of grandchildren. Elderly women help also in decision-making and daily chores. While the majority of women continue to live with their families several factors have made this ideal problematic.

Many Goans have left their ancestral homes in rural areas and moved to growing towns to avail of better educational facilities for their children. They have left behind their aged parents in their ancestral homes to look after themselves. Goans, particularly from Christian community have also been out-migrating in significant numbers in post-colonial times. They have been migrating to different parts of the globe to the Americas, Europe, Australia, and New Zealand or for shorter periods to the Middle East. This migration has been necessitated by lack of employment facilities, the desire for better standard of living, better educational facilities elsewhere or as more recent trends in migration to New Zealand, Australia and Canada have shown a 'better future for the children'. This future often does not include the ageing parents or elder members of the family who are left behind in their own homes or institutionalised in retirement homes. At other times children who have migrated have taken their healthy/active mother with them leaving behind an old infirm father in a 'home'(RIW, 2002).

All elderly women in Goa do not live with their immediate family. Some live by themselves while others in the company of a maid or a neighbour who keeps company at night. From a survey conducted among 25 women in the fourth age group: 8 live by themselves with a maid for company not far from other members of the family, 7 live with one of the married sons, his wife and children, 3 woman live with an unmarried daughter, 1 with a bachelor son, 1 unmarried older woman lives with a another unmarried sibling, 1 has the company of a nephew and his family who live with her in her house and 4 live with their spouses. They belong to upper and middle-income group. About 6 of the women interviewed are financially dependent on their children, 2 depend on their spouses. Others have their own sources of income from properties or pension of their dead husbands. Three derived income from business started by their husbands and five were professionals who receive pensions, have savings and family property. They spend their time performing various tasks at home, knitting, reading, social work, watching TV, praying, working in some activities, going out for long walks or looking after grandchildren. All are literate and six have received higher education.

Majority of elderly women in Goa in the fourth age group are illiterate, a small number know only to read and write. The incidence of widowhood among women aged 75 years and above is quite high in Goa as in Kerala (Gulati *et al.*, 1999). From the above-mentioned survey it was found that out of 25 women, 18 are widows and they belong to the fourth age group. This incidence is high because of age difference between husband and wife. As in other parts of India there is age difference between spouses (on average females are at least five years younger than males) and unlike in the past women today in Goa have a greater life expectancy due to better medical facilities.

As they advance in age, women's dependence especially physical dependence on other members of the family increases. This takes a lot time and energy of the family members. At other times the mental conditions of the elderly women—confused state of mind or irritable nature can contribute to domestic conflicts.

Sense of isolation is another major problem in Goa among elderly women of all strata of the society. Increasingly, there are cases where elderly women who live within the family are left to themselves for greater part of the day as other members of the family go to work. The situation of elderly women depends also on the place where they live—in urban or rural areas. The condition of those who live in the village on their own is apparently better in some aspects than those in urban areas. People in the villages are more friendly and supportive. The elderly in the villages have the company and comfort of other relatives living nearby or neighbours who often lend a helping hand.

The number of women in retirement homes in Goa is progressing. Many complain about the need to have better homes for the elderly as if that is the best solution for the older people. Recently, a Goan gentleman living Europe who has his mother in Canada living with another sibling and is planning to send his mother to a 'retirement home' in Goa wrote, "Old people are very sensitive and feel they are being dumped by their ungrateful children but often it is to their best". Goa has almost 38 'homes' most of them in Tiswadi, Bardez and Salcete talukas to cater to the needs of all sections of population. But the conditions in majority of these homes are dismal.

A glance at the many retirement homes in Goa that we have visited in the last 3 years reveal that the majority of elders living in these 'homes' are women. Out of 73 residents in a 'home' in Tiswadi taluka, 46 were women. Most 'homes' have more women than men. There are 12 'homes' only for women as compared to 5 'homes' only for men (RIW, 2002). What explains this large population of institutionalised older women?

From the study conducted by Research Institute for Women, we have gathered that women residents particularly married and widows were forced to move away from their own homes on account of strained relations with other members mainly with daughters-in-law, unmarried sisters-in-law and lack of domestic help in the house to look after the old. Very few women have moved from their own homes willingly. In a "Retirement Home" in Bardez taluka out of 19 married women residents, 12 had their children living in Goa and 3 had children living abroad. In another 'home' in the same taluka out of 12 women residents, 10 had children in Goa. Yet in another 'home' out of 14 married women residents, 6 had children in Goa while 5 had children living abroad. There are cases of strained relations between husband and wife after a long married life. At other times, women who outlive their husbands in the third and fourth age group have often no independent source of income to support them and they go to the 'homes' not to be a burden to others in the family. There are cases when elderly illiterate mothers have been sent to the 'home' because not being literate their educated children and grandchildren consider them an embarrassment to have them in their houses. They are considered as old fashioned and irrelevant in the present day scenario. Some women whose children have migrated and are unable to live alone also go to the retirement 'homes'.

Furthermore, many women who have worked for a large part of their lives as domestic staff in Goa and outside in places such as Bombay, Pune, Calcutta, Karachi or Gwalior living with/working for other people's families have moved into 'homes' when they could no longer work. They are usually not married, have no one to look after them and are often seen as a burden by their employers. Sometimes constraints of living space in urban areas make matters difficult for the employers. In Goa, there is also another group of women—the unmarried elderly who have no one to look after them and prefer to go to the 'homes' when they are no longer able to take care of themselves. Majority of women in these 'homes' from middle-income group are Christians. Until recently there were no separate homes for Hindus, Hindu women were reluctant to go to 'homes' where people of other community lived. Besides the joint families took care of their elderly, this does not mean that they do not have problems like their Christian counterparts but somehow they are forced to reconcile to their fate.

As already mentioned a few women go to the retirement homes willingly. From the interview conducted among the resident of these retirement 'homes' we have realised that majority of women would like to stay in their own milieu where they have spent major part of their life. At older age, it is difficult for them to live in new surroundings, make new friends and neighbours. Retirement 'homes' give a feeling of rejection and the conditions in many of them are dismal in terms of facilities and atmosphere. Many families do not keep in touch with their relatives once they are taken to the retirement 'homes'.

Conditions in residential institutions should have been like a home but it has been noticed that most 'homes' resemble more like a hospital/dormitories with its rows of bed rather then a home. The residents have no privacy and facilities. Often they have to keep their belongings under the bed and they do not even have a table or chair all for themselves. They have to share accommodation with others and there is restriction on their movements. 'Homes' run by the State do not even have a telephone through which the residents can keep contact with their families.

## Health Status of Elderly

In post-colonial times, women in Goa are living longer then men due to improvement in socio-economic conditions and availability of health facilities. Besides, in case of married ones there is always age difference between husbands and wife. The custom that, women should be younger than their husband is still taken into consideration when selecting partners, especially in case of arranged marriages.

During the colonial period mortality rate among women was high due to health problems and lack of medical facilities. Women married very young and spent a considerable part of their adult life pregnant or nursing. They suffered higher level of infectious diseases. Along with poorer nutrition, lack of knowledge of asepsis at the time of delivery contributed to the adult female excess of death over males throughout childbearing ages. Adult female excess of death over males was largely from maternal mortality, tuberculosis and malaria.

Child bearing was a difficult process in Goa as still is in many developing countries (Gracias, 1994). Large numbers of women still die in some parts of south Asia during pregnancy and childbirth. High mortality rate among women in Goa during pregnancy in the earlier centuries was the result of the conditions surrounding the pregnant mother before during and after delivery. Delivery throughout the colonial period and even sometime afterwards was conducted at home. A small section resorted to the help of doctors for delivery. The birth was attended by a *Dai* or Voijin (midwife), who had scanty knowledge of hygiene. Lack of transport and poverty also prevented people in need of medical facilities to seek the help of doctors in towns. Furthermore, as mentioned earlier in Goa girls particularly from lower strata married early, even before they completed their growth. Poor body built and statures were major causes of obstetric risks. Women had large number of children due to religious influence. High mortality rate led to economic necessity of bearing many children so that some may survive to provide much needed manual labour in agriculture. More births were needed to ensure surviving adults when the parents become old. These are some of the factors that contributed to maternity deaths (*ibid.* 61).

Girls due to lack of care and diseases did not survive for long. Males were better looked after in the early days of birth and very often survived diseases. Pronounced preference for sons led to poorer feeding and neglect of daughters. This could be due to lack of education and other factors.

However, the census report shows excess of females over males in the first half of twentieth century in Goa. In 1900 there were 2,75,973 females for 2,25,825 males (Census, 1900). By 1931 the number of females had increased to 3,00,572 (Census, 1931). The highest number of females per 1,000 males was in 1950. In this year there were 1,128 females for 1,000 males (Census, 1950). The census of 1960 showed a slight decline with 1,066 females for 1,000 males. The ratio in favour of the females particularly in the early decades of 20th century was due to variety of factors. Among these out migration was an important one. Large number of Goans migrated during this period to British India, British and Portuguese Africa and later to the Middle East. Generally they left behind their wives and mothers.

Although, women in Goa today have higher life expectancy they do not always enjoy good health. Many have age related ailments. Women's health sees changes proceeding and following menopause much before they reach old age. Many women sail through this period with much ease and without any health problems but for others these changes brings striking hormonal peculiarities. Reduced ovarian hormonal level sometimes plays key role in osteoporosis, cardiovascular diseases, loss of bone and muscle. Menopause brings a variety of psychological changes too as result of reduced ovarian functions.

Failing eyesight, impaired hearing, arthritis, loss of memory, teeth falls and fractures are common among many old women in the fourth age group. Some of these conditions restrict social interaction, leads to isolation and sometimes-even depression. Depression and sense of isolation is common among the elderly women in Goa. Other common health problems are hypertension, diabetics, spondulitis, cancer, urinary infections and constipation. Urinary incontinence is also common in women as in men.

Among 8 women in the fourth age group who were interviewed for this paper, two were overweight, one had a stroke and has survived to reach 91 years, and 3 have arthritis/ osteoporosis. One has been diagnosed with irreversible Alzameirhs disease; one suffers from Parkinson for several years and one from regular bouts of depression. Majority of them live with their families.

Neither the government nor private organisations have paid enough attention to the health care of the elderly. There are no Gerontology centres to care of them. With a few exception majority of retirement 'homes' in Goa do not have even a nursing home/ward in its premises. However, some government-managed homes have doctors attached who are available on call and nursing staff who work on shifts.

Unlike in some other places, in Goa women do not go for regular health check-ups. There are no mandatory health checks and tests for older women. Women are reluctant to visit a physician unless they are ill. There is lack of information about medical facilities available to elder women besides majority of them cannot afford costly health checks and tests. Even a few who can afford do not make use of the facilities available to them in towns and cities. Many women being uneducated are ignorant of the possible ailments related to the old age and therefore not in a position to take any preventive steps. Women living in villages have to come to towns to avail of the facilities. At other times due to their advanced age and ill health they depend on their relatives to travel.

Elderly women in Goa lead a sedentary life and rarely exercise. As one woman who was interviewed said "exercising is not part of our way of life, women do not go out alone for walks" Regular exercise is not a part of women's routine, exercise which could help control arthritis, reduce wait, control diabetes, cholesterol and cardiovascular disease. Majority of women are either overweight or underweight and take no measures to control their weight by regular exercise and diet.

On account of various ailments and age, the elderly need to have a special diet. The diet depends on economic conditions of the person, custom and the place where they live. If the woman lives alone she can have a special diet that may not be easy to prepare if she lives with her family. On the other hand, there is also tendency to neglect the diet while living alone. As result of their financial dependence in many cases nutritious food is begrudged to them. In some cases nutritious food is provide to the grandchildren in the family and the least nutritious to the aged. Diet of majority of elderly women in Goa is poor. It is rich in carbohydrates and lacking in proteins, calcium, milk, dark leafy vegetables and fruits. The diet is poor due to poor knowledge and financial constraints. There are also cases when certain types of food may not agree and lead to other complication.

A few Suggestions that could help the elderly women in Goa :

- Majority of women in the third and fourth age group still live with their families. They need attention and love. There is need to retrain them in new skills suitable for their age. A second career for active elderly women needs to be studied. The services of older women who are active could be constructively used as caregivers. Older women are sources of wisdom, knowledge and experience. These could be used for the benefit of the society and to ensure their well-being as well as of their families. There is need to make the elderly self-sufficient.

- There is need for 24 hours service on the lines of child help to help the elderly in need of counselling and particularly for those who are harshly treated by their families.
- Since caring for the very old is often physically and emotionally stressful, community support must be organised to help families to cope. Self-help groups and voluntary organisations on the lines of Stichting Dienstverlering in the Netherlands (Krishnaraj, 1999) or Misericordias in Portugal should reach the elderly, destitute old women, disabled, emotionally affected women so as to give some relief to the families who have been looking after them full time day care centres, night care centres, buddy services involving the young, volunteer networks and such creative responses will go a long way in making the care of the aged more manageable.
- Goa has many big houses in the villages that are closed. These houses if available could be converted in day care centres where elder women could spend their time constructively or just relaxing with others and sharing a meal. Weekly medical, counselling and other services could be provided for elder women in these centres. In Portugal *Santa Casa Misericordia,* a social welfare organisation for instance provides day home care for bedridden and night care for the lonely and isolated (*A Vos das Misericordias* 2000, 2001). In Netherlands, there are private companies that organise the care of the elderly.
- A pool of nurses could be made available in Goa itself

to those in need of home care instead of getting them all the way from outside the state. This also would provide employment to many women.

- Development programmes to educate the elderly to facilitate ageing, cope with final stages of life, bereavement in the family especially of a spouse or a grown up offspring, isolation and death need to be organised.
- Women in the third and fourth stage of life should be encouraged to go for bi-annual health checks free of cost. For this purpose they should be provided with necessary information where such facilities are available.
- Special seats for the aged may be the first six seats should be reserved in public transport system. State is providing a few facilities and subsidies for the aged but these are not sufficient to meet the minimum needs of elder women. Free medical check-up and other medical facilities should be made available to the public.
- While the ideal situation would be to keep the elder women within their own surroundings there are times when it is not possible to have them at home. As they may not be able to live alone, have problems with other members of the family or they may not have financial possibilities to maintain themselves. Since the conditions of the majority of the retirement homes are not satisfactory, there is need to improve these homes to make them look like a home rather then a hospital ward.

**REFERENCES**

A. Voz das Misericordias a monthly journal published by Santa Casa da Misericordia, Lisboa December 2000, January,2001 and February 2001 issues.

Census of India Reports of 1900, 1931, 1950.

Dessai Murli 1999: 'Ageing of Women in Post-Menopausal Stage: Need for Intervention', *Economic and Political Weekly,* October 30- November 5.

Gracias Fatima da Silva 1994: *Health and Hygiene in Colonial Goa,1510-1961,* New Delhi, Concept.

Gracias Fatima da Silva 2000: 'Goans away from Goa—Migration to Middle East' Lusophonies Asiatiques, Asiatiques en Lusophonies in *Lusotopie,* Paris.

Gulati Leela and S. Irudaya Rajan 1999: 'The Added Years—Elderly in India and Kerala', *Economic and Political Weekly,* October 30-November 5.

Krishnaraj Maithreyi 1999: 'Ageing Women in a Welfare State-Cracks in the Utopia', *Economic and Political Weekly,* October 30-November 5.

(RIW) Research Institute for Women 2002: *Age and Wisdom Undervalued: An Inquiry into the Social Process of Ageing in Goa at the Turn of the Third Millennium* (A Report), RIW, Goa.

16

# A GENDERED PERSPECTIVE OF THE HEALTH OF THE DIFFERENTLY ABLED AND THE DISABLED

*Melsa Vas Monteiro*

The Rights of the Differently-Abled (DA) and the Disabled (D) are protected by The Persons With Disabilities (Equal Opportunities, Protection of Rights and Full Participation) Act, 1995. It was enacted by Parliament to give effect to the Proclamation made on the Full Participation and Equality of the People with Disabilities in the Asian and Pacific Region meeting convened by ESC for Asia and Pacific Region held at Beijing in December 1992, to which India was a signatory. The Act came into effect from January 1996.

The State of Goa has fulfilled the recommendations of the above Act by :

- Establishing the State level Committee for the Welfare of Handicapped Persons with the Minister for Social Welfare as the Chairperson, 10 Official Members and 6 Non-Official Members;
- Constituting the State Coordination Committee with 16 Ex-officio Members and 6 others;
- Constituting the State Executive Committee with 12 Ex-officio Members and 6 others;
- Setting up a District Disability and Rehabilitation Centre (DDRC).

The Directorate of Social Welfare, which attends to the needs of the Differently-Abled and the Disabled compiled and published a Report on the Survey of Persons with Disability in Goa at a Seminar they organised on the theme "Equal Rights of and Welfare Measures for the Disabled" in 1997. It is learnt that the information collected then has not been updated in the past five years.

**Who are the Differently-Abled and the Disabled?**

The Professional/Official classification of disabilities given by the Directorate of Social Welfare in their Survey of Persons with Disability in Goa—1997 lists the following disabilities :

Orthopaedically Handicapped (OH); Visually Handicapped (VH); Hearing Handicapped (HH); Mentally Retarded (MR); Multiple Handicapped (ML); Medically Handicapped (MH); and Leprosy Cured (LC). People deemed fitting into these categories merit the benefits offered to the DA/D in the State of Goa.

However, different definitions of the word 'disability' are available depending on the source. Lay persons committed to the cause of the DA and D encounter many cases, specially in the rural areas that clamour attention, but do not appear to fit into the categories described above. Their helplessness is compounded as information and guidance is not easily available at their level. Responsible persons in the Agencies within their reach are often not sufficiently well-informed or trained or motivated and hence they remain indifferent to the genuine needs of the disabled.

Worse is the position of 'low status groups': illiterate, semi-illiterate, uninformed, misinformed, steeped in superstitions living in the rural, suburban areas and in settlements in urban pockets. The education of these vulnerable groups is neglected. Consequently they are denied opportunities to empower the differently abled to avail of their rights for their advancement. This is gross indifference to the Rights of the DA/D by a large section of the Goan Society.

It becomes necessary to cite some of such cases:

- A child in a Middle School repeating a class for two years (she/he has come up to this level as promotion to the Higher Class in the Primary School each year is compulsory). In the case of the girl-child, her schooling will probably be discontinued. What will her future be?
- A young woman turned neurotic because of adjustment problems (ill-treatment) in the house of the in-laws. It can well be imagined what kind of treatment will be meted out to her?
- Village 'simpletons', nick-named 'enddo', 'goui', 'pixi', liberally used to run errands, work in houses, gardens, properties, paid a pittance and booted out (even featured in Goa's tiatrs). Who is responsible to restore their rights?
- A young girl with oral deformity (cleft lip and palate). Is her dignity protected?

**Where are the Differently Abled?**

Are all the disabled officially acknowledged (accounted for)?

Any attempts to reach beyond statistics must be based on REALITY. Hence, it becomes necessary to spare a cursory glance at Statistics compiled by the Directorate of Social Welfare.

**Number of disabled persons in Goa (1997)**

*(No update available)*

| | *Male* | *Female* | *Total* |
|---|---|---|---|
| OH | 3114 | 1846 | 4960 |
| VH | 673 | 548 | 1221 |
| HH | 811 | 714 | 1525 |
| MR | 902 | 726 | 1628 |
| MH | 330 | 189 | 519 |
| ML | 185 | 127 | 312 |
| LC | 71 | 27 | 98 |
| Total | 6086 | 4177 | 10263 |

| Population of Goa (1991 Census) | |
|---|---|
| Male: | 5,94,790 |
| Female: | 5,75,003 |
| Total: | 11,69,793 |
| (2001 Census) | |
| Male: | 6,85,617 |
| Female: | 6,58,681 |
| Total: | 13,43,998 |

**Do these above figures depict the REALITY?**

According to the UN Programme of Action concerning disabled persons in countries like India, at least one person in ten is DA/D by physical, mental or sensory impairment. Separate statistics of Differently-Abled and Disabled afflicted with AIDS/HIV+ve are not easily available. It is learnt that the Central Government Statistical Cell in Goa is in the process of finalising a detailed compilation.

The first step towards reaching out has necessarily to identify and locate the differently abled in various parts of Goa.

**What Are the Facilities Offered Presently in Goa?**

- There are 10 organisations that offer educational facilities for the disabled children. Of these, 3 offer residential facilities. Health care is part of their programme.
- In the Homes run by the Public Assistance Department for the poor and destitute, a small number of differently abled and disabled are admitted.
- Medical facilities are available (along with the general public) at Rural Centres, the 2 District Hospitals and the Goa Medical College.
- Special Medical facilities are available at the Institute of Psychiatry and Human Behaviour (IPHB). They have facilities for IQ testing and A Child Guidance Centre for children below 13.
- The G.M.C. has a special programme of Rural Camps for the Disabled in 9 Talukas at 10 Centres where the Faculty Team visit each Centre once a month. The statistics of services provided in the past year are given below :

The Statistics of the District Disability and Rehabilitation Centre, Goa (DDRC) for September 2001-October 2002 states the following :

| | Males | | Females | |
|---|---|---|---|---|
| | (Below 14) | (Above 14) | (Below 14) | (Above 14) |
| MR | 62 | 109 | 46 | 85 |
| HH | 117 | 111 | 63 | 114 |
| OH | 82 | 214 | 56 | 126 |
| VH | 33 | 154 | 20 | 189 |
| Total | 294 | 588 | 185 | 514 |

- N.G.O.'s like Sangath and others provide IQ testing and Counselling facilities.

**Societal Environment and Its Impact on the Differently-abled/Disabled**

Goa is acknowledged as socio-culturally advanced and a highly literate State. Hence, the recognition and acceptance of the DA/D as full-fledged citizens with equal rights, should be a foregone conclusion. Is it so in reality? Efforts by NGO's and the Government have contributed significantly to attitudinal changes in favour of the DA/D. More people recognise the rights of the DA/D and are sympathetic towards their cause.

But quite a large section of society still seems to believe that the DA/D are an unavoidable burden to be dragged along (not clear by whom) and their attitude is consequently condescending. Besides, in many sections of Society, a disability is considered a 'punishment' or a 'curse' or a result of 'evil eye'. Superstitious beliefs play a forceful role in thwarting the effects of Awareness Motivation Programmes. These are extremely biased against the female. Blocks still exist specially within the family of the DA/D. What are the causes of these blocks?

- Lack of awareness Misconceptions, Confusion
- Fear of being labelled, rejected Overprotection, Abandonment

The impact of this attitude and behaviour on the

Differently-Abled and Disabled person is disastrous, specially on the female. The person feels unwanted, guilty, lacks self worth whereas she/he needs to be accepted as a person, needs much love, care and assurance. The lack of these or on the contrary, discrimination and bias give rise to psychological imbalances and add to the already impaired health.

The health problems of each group of the DA/D are different and need corresponding treatment for holistic health promotion. Persons with Physical and Sensory impairment can observe, compare, rationalise and realise their limitations, privations and dependence on others in different ways. Unless properly counselled, they will feel negated and react in bursts of unreasonable behaviour, which most times is not understood by even the family members. They should be motivated, guided and encouraged to develop their latent talents to find fulfillment in activities they are capable of.

Another sphere that poses problems for the adolescents is their sexual development and natural desires. Their disability becomes a block in building healthy relationships with the opposite sex. Special education by professionals is a must in this important phase of their lives.

Those Mentally Retarded, whether mildly or moderately, will face problems similar to those in the above category, while those with severe and profound mental retardation, are generally physically strong. Their behaviour is spontaneous and unpredictable. Being unable to distinguish the importance of protection of vital parts of the body or to judge the impact and consequences of their action, they can cause injury to self and others. Hence they need constant vigilance by capable persons.

## Position of Differently-Abled/Disabled Women, Girl-Children

Today when women are perceived as "commodities" to meet the needs of others, specially "desires" of men, a woman or girl-child with disabilities is much more vulnerable to rejection and ridicule and these disadvantages impede her chances to overcome the disability with proper health-care, although this is her right. She is hidden away in her home or other 'homes' and is abused physically, emotionally and sexually. She is considered a 'burden'. She is made to work hard in the home despite her disability as her prospects of marriage are poor. Women and grown up girls shoulder the entire burden of caring for the disabled, specially if the person needs constant care as in the case of severe physical deformity and multiple mental retardation like Down Syndrome, Cerebral Palsy, Multiple Sclerosis, Paraplegia, Torticollis, Osteoarthritis, Parkinsonism, Alzheimer's, etc. In many cases she herself is mildly or moderately disabled. The women/girls are under psychological stress and need health care themselves. They are entitled to it, but this aspect is totally neglected. They do not assert their rights as they are socially conditioned to accept such situations as their fate. Thus, the 'culture of gender discrimination' is strengthened and perpetuated.

Again sensitive disabilities of the reproductive system like infertility and genital malformation are stigmas. The treatment meted out to infertile women is well known, but not highlighted. It often leads women to commit suicide instead of seeking corrective medical intervention, which would have in all probability remedied her condition and resulted in fulfillment of her motherhood. The recent tragedy of the celebrated athlete, Prathima Gaonkar is a proof.

The situation in Goa keeps improving because of advocacy and empowerment Programmes by Women's Groups.

## The Middle Aged and Elderly

About thirty years ago, and more so in the earlier times, in most villages of Goa barring the 'higher status class', the untrained mid-wife guided by her inborn talent (hat-gunn) and her past experiences, delivered babies and attended to both the new-born and the mother using means and methods best known to her to face the situation she encountered. In these circumstances any non-visible defects went undetected and if they were, like cleft lip, were kept a close guarded secret, specially if they were females. Hence, today there are a number of women, victims of disabilities, denied their rights and suffering indignities.

Besides, there are cases of Dementia, Parkinsonism,

Alzheimer's, etc. who, specially if they are women, do not get the health care they urgently need.

**Rehabilitation Programme**

What does it imply?

- Restoration of the fullest physical, mental, social, vocational and economic usefulness of which the given disabled person is capable. It includes all measures aimed at reducing the impact enabling her/him to achieve certain goals.

The Rehabilitated Disabled person should enjoy:

– Independence with protection of human rights;
– Social integration and adaptation of the environment with family and community involvement;
– A better quality of life attaining usefulness and satisfaction.

**Recommendations**

The following are urgent needs of the Differently-Abled and Disabled to obtain their dues:

- An all-inclusive Handbook with indicators to identify and categorise DA/D.
- The registering of such cases at least at the Panchayat level could be made mandatory.
- A competent mechanism to identify and locate all the DA/D. Village Panchayats could be associated with this work. A thorough periodic update is a must.
- An updated Directory of Government agencies and schemes for the DA/D giving clear instructions on how to obtain them. It should include a list of NGO's in Goa with types of services they offer.
- A mechanism for dissemination of all the above information (use of multiple media).
- A programme for the education and sensitization, specially of the uninformed/misinformed in the rural, sub-urban and urban areas as the focus.

- Establishment of a Centre in each Taluka for the health care of the Differently-Abled and Disabled with professionals, trained counsellors and primary health care workers, different for each category, offering regular services at least once a week. A one window source for funding could be part of this Unit. The health care and counselling of the family members (caretakers) of the disabled should be part of this programme. A Referral System to various Hospitals and other Specialised Service Institutions needs to be established.
- Establishment of a Training cum Production Centre in each Taluka where the DA of each category can be trained and given employment in production work under the Schemes for self-employment.
- Creating an Environment of Accessibility and facilities in Public Utility Buildings to enable the DA/D to function independently.
- Well planned and vigorously conducted Special Awareness Programmes for the affirmation of DA/D girl-children and women with the help of Women's Organisations and other NGO's.
- Formation of a State-level Audit Team.

**Some Additional Proposals and Recommendations**

***Caritas, Goa***

Reflecting the various aspects of health, particularly with regard to the handicap, we would like to put forth a few proposals, recommendations to be addressed by all the concerned persons and institutions.

- We need to stress the urgent need for a holistic health programme of rehabilitation on behalf of the disabled.
- It would be pertinent to integrate disability prevention and rehabilitation into primary health care strategies.
- Malnutrition and disease in pregnancy and early childhood are the major causes of disability. The

*contd.*

*contd.*

primary health care workers backed by training and linking them to government health services can significantly reduce the incidence and severity of disabilities *e.g.* Merely supplying vitamin A can prevent thousands of children from going blind, not doing so amounts to a crime.

- Nutritional education through practical methods can prevent low-birth weight babies who are more prone to be blind, deaf-mute, mentally retarded and crippled.
- All efforts must be made to rectify defects or reduce the disability of a child born with multiple congenital infirmities.
- The government must provide medical treatment, including corrective surgery for the physical rehabilitation of the disabled.
- Be it in family, school or society various programmes need to be organised since the disabled are the ones who most need stimulation and involvement.
- Designing all public utility offices/buildings wherein the disabled can manage their affairs by themselves. Creating an Environment of Accessibility.
- Educational institutions should seriously deal with matters relating to relationships, sex-education, gift of life, etc.
- In the State Education Policy, aspecial section to deal with the needs and problems of the handicap should be immediately taken up. Also a special curriculum for all special schools in Goa is of urgent need.
- Compulsory education for all physically handicapped children and facilities for higher education to those who have aptitude for it is demanded.
- To provide vocational training to the trainable and then provide employment to the employable. Also they should be encouraged to undertake self-employment enterprises.

*The society owes the disabled help. This help is not simply a question of sympathy or charity. It is a moral duty. It is a question of social justice.*

# NOVEL PERSPECTIVES OF OLD HEALTH SYSTEMS

# 17

# WOMEN AND INDIGENOUS HEALTH CARE IN GOA

*Bernadette Gomes*

Indigenous Medicine, known as 'Gamvto vokot' in Goa, includes all remedies using plant and animal parts. It also includes other practices for recovering health such as removal of evil eye (dixttichem), and driving away evil spirits that make a person sick (varyachem). 'Ghorguti vokot' stands for all the home remedies provided by family members (mainly women) to their kinsfolk and neighbours. They are the first remedies to be administered in case of illness. This paper will take a look at health care in a traditional setting. The focus will be on the role women have played in providing:

(*a*) Nutrition for the family.
(*b*) Health care and cures.
(*c*) Pre-natal and Post-natal care.

## Belief and Illness

Among the Kunbi community, from where data for this paper has been used, there is a belief that women have a larger potential in causing illness to others in the community. They can cause evil eye more frequently as compared to men. When people die under tragic circumstances in the prime of their life, they become malevolent spirits. Women here too, are more vicious compared to their male counterparts. They can cause illness to living members in the community. Ironically women have also been the major providers of health care in the community.

## Women and Indigenous Medicine

In order to understand women's role in indigenous health care, we have to begin with women's work in a traditional setting. The jobs they do are—Cooking, cleaning the house, cultivation, selling fish and vegetables, clearing land (bhenop), working as wage labourers. Out of the various jobs that they do, clearing land, collecting firewood and cultivation, brings them in close physical contact with the land. They are closely involved with the flora and fauna of the land. Incidentally it is the women who are mainly involved in these occupations. Thus their participation in the traditional labour structure offers them and excellent opportunity for collecting roots, barks, herbs, which may be needed in the event of an illness.

Women have developed a culture of collecting medicines for the family. In the course of their work, they are alert to their larger role as providers of health care to the family. Thus while clearing land, cutting firewood, women also collect roots, leaves and other plant parts simultaneously. This is a deep-rooted practice often done unconsciously by women.

Some women are acknowledged as having the healing touch 'haat gunn'. Such women dispense medicine to the villagers. They are called as the 'voktamkarn'. A man would be called a 'voktamkar'. The 'haat gunn' is one of the important criteria to determine a woman's status as 'voktamkarn' or mere knowledge of medicines is not enough. Once a person has been identified as a victim of evil eye, it is removed through a ritual. Here too women are mainly involved. They are called as the 'dixttikarn'. Though there are men in both cases, the number of women far outnumber men.

## Sentinels of Nutrition and Health

In a traditional household, women shoulder all culinary responsibilities. They are the sole providers of meals to the family. A child's first nutrition comes from the mother's body itself, as breast milk. The mother continues to be the source of good food for her family for the rest of her working life. This is not merely through her cooking abilities. Traditionally, Kunbis have practised a strict diet regime varying with the seasons. Foods available during a season are believed to be suited for that period. Also certain food is avoided. For example healthy foods are avoided in summer, but eaten generously during the winter. The people have developed a belief system, which is enforced and executed through the women folk of the community. A mother cooks the foods appropriate during the season, for her family. Seasonal diets are believed to be important to maintain health.

The high degree of importance given to food as a source of good health can be illustrated from the following:—When a family member, be it an adult or a child first utters the words "I am not feeling well!" the mother's first question always is, "what did you eat?". The question is significant because it is directly related to food. It implies that food is believed to be of prime importance in maintaining health. It follows that the providers of good food, namely women are crucial to the health care programme of the community. We can conclude that the women of the community become the sentinels of the community's health some of the good items used in their daily diet may also be put to multiple use.

Certain foods are used as medicines as well. If a person suffers from constipation, he is given generous helpings of papaya. To avoid colds during the monsoon a sweet gruel made with *moong* (a lentel) is eaten generously. Mild stomach upsets are treated with *hing* (asofetida) and *jeera* (cumin). Women with their culinary responsibilities possess knowledge of a wide number of recipies, which are beneficial for common ailments, (*e.g.* constipation, diarrhoea, colds). Thus 'ghorguti vokot' begins with household foods and condiments. These are the first remedies administered in the case of illness. Once again we find that preliminary medication also comes from the women themselves.

'Ganvti vokod' or other herbal remedies provided by the 'voktamkarn', or 'voktamkar' formed the second line of treatment. Finally, allopathy or 'bailem vokod' is sought as a cure. Following the line of treatment, we see that maintenance of good health began with good food and a strict diet regime. Good food began with the women of the household. The preliminary remedies also began with food items, which were also provided by women. Therefore we can conclude that family health began at the hands of women in a traditional set-up.

## Women, Childbirth and Childcare

In a traditional set-up, childbirth, childcare and knowledge of birth control were the domain of women. Childbirth was conducted entirely by women. The special birth attendants were called as 'voijinn'. They took responsibility of delivery 'partho' and the confinement and recovery of the mother 'baloutin'. Along with the female members of the family 'voijinns' supervised the first 30 days of the mother's confinements. A 'voijinn' single-handedly managed the delivery of a child. Other family members merely assisted her. No men were ever involved in the 'partho' or post-natal care.

The 'Voijinn' had special knowledge of the following :

Diet restrictions and special foods for the pregnant mother.

Good/bad sleeping positions, depending on position of foetus.

Methods to check the position of the foetus.

Special massager with hands and feet to alter position of foetus (in case of a breach baby).

Pressures to be exerted in difficult deliveries.

List of antiseptics, douches, bio-sealants, to be used for vaginal tears after delivery.

Massage for the infant.

Special herbal drinks charms for infant, to prevent colic gas, evil eye.

Special diet for the mother for the first 30 days after delivery 'jitem'.

Special sleeping positions for facilitating lactation, preventing inflammation of breasts, and muscle cramps.

## The Scenario Today

Almost all 'voijinns' and 'voktamkarns' today would be more than 70 years of age. They are not actively involved in providing health care. They do however provide valuable advice to pregnant women and other sick persons on certain do's and don'ts. In some villages they assist the doctors from the primary health centres in conducting a delivery. They are also storehouses of valuable folk gynaecological knowledge, and traditional remedies.

## Plan of Action

At this juncture a one point plan of action can be suggested. The Government of Goa through the auspices of the Centre for Women's studies or the State Commission for Women can be requested to institute a scholarship of not less than two years duration, together exhaustive information on the following:

Annual Nutritional Pattern
Folk-Gynaecology
Anti-Fertility Plants
Pre-natal, Post-natal Care.

**Maintenance of Good Health**

| *Degree of Importance* | *Source* | *Controlled By* |
|---|---|---|
| Primary | Food/Nutrition | Women |
| Secondary | Home Remedies (Ghorgutt Vokot) | Women |
| Tertiary | Herbal Remedies (Ganvti Vokod) | Women and Men |
| Ultimate | Allopathy (Bailed Vokod) | Women and Men |

# 18

# STRENGTHENING THE SCOPE OF HOMEOPATHIC CARE IN GOA

*Usha Salelkar*

Homeopathy was unheard of in the 60's as it was banned in Goa due to Portuguese Regime. However the policy in the late ex-Prime Minister Mr. Morarji Desai's Government, saw the introduction of Homeopathy and Ayurveda in all states of the country in the year 70's. Goa however did not feel the need of such an introduction till 1978 when the Government of Goa introduced the first clinic in Goa in Panaji under the Directorate of Health Services. The author of this paper was appointed as the first homeopathic physician there. The following is the narration of some of the authors experiences and recommendations.

To bring up the clinic, I had to face, number of difficulties. It was an obstacle race from the very beginning. Pressures faced included the type of setting. The clinic was in a dilapidated state, with no proper ventilation. It was unhygienic with facilities for privacy to talk to the female patients. It certainly did not invite many patients in the beginning. Homeopathic Medicines were also not provided due to official lapses. For example, tenders for the same medicines were not advertised for 6 months. In those days Homeopathic medicines were not available in Goa and we had to rely only on medicines which we bought from Bombay to start private clinic or that we asked patients to get from Belgaum or Bombay.

It took nearly one year for news of this clinic to reach the ears of other patients only by way of mouth. There was not much awareness through any other media. Slowly and steadily the clinic was visited especially by residents of other states who were aware of this form of medication other than the local Goan community. It was only after 3 to 4 years persons with chronic cases would queue up at the clinic. It then became difficult for me to handle the number of patients all alone. People had to take appointments so that they would not go back disappointed from the North end of Goa to the South. I made repeated requests to the Directors, Secretaries, written and personal to increase the staff and budget for the clinic. However, my file had increased in its volume with no effect.

Ten years later, under the scheme 'Rural Development' one post of Homeopathic Physician was introduced in a rural area namely Pernem. During those days the urgent need was in the cities, as people were aware of this form of medicine. People from Vasco made a request to the Minister to invite me at least once a week to the clinic which was of urgent need in the area as no other Homeopathic doctor was available during those days. The Pernem doctor was asked to go to Margao twice a week. The government however did not increase the number of posts.

It used to be very strenuous for us. It became very difficult for us to manage such a large number of patients in Goa. The lapses in the decisions by the Government have today given me the opportunity to come forward to voice my experiences today.

After twenty two years I was promoted as the Senior Physician in this clinic *i.e.* only 1 ½ years prior to my retirement without creating a new post. The position today in the 21st Century remains the same only in Goa. However, the only improvement we have today, is the introduction of homeopathic medicines in a few pharmacies in Margao, Mapusa and Panaji by local pharmacist.

We can very well compare today's development in other states, which are well advanced. There are 20,000 dispensaries, 300 hospitals, 200 teaching institutions and 300 drug manufacturing units all over India. Most of states like Karnataka, Andhra Pradesh, Bihar, Delhi, have a separate homeopathic directorate with deputy directors and a number of medical officers too. Now post-graduate courses also are started in many states.

It is important for us to awaken and make people conscious of the slackening development of this branch of medicine in Goa. Occasions like these help us exchange our views and make our representations more forceful. The development in this field is not for a single individual but for the teeming millions.

Homeopathy is a wonderful science effective in certain conditions like allergies and other chronic ailments. As a young girl, I was going through a severe problem of constant allergic colds for 15 years and no allopathic doctor, nor surgery would help. I was even taken to Portugal for treatment. But it was to no avail. Then when I went to Bombay for higher studies I was healed by a homeopath, the father of one of my friends. Since then I have believed in the efficacy of this stream of medicine.

It might be pertinent to note that after I finished my training as a homeopath, I worked as a Junior Medical Officer at the Goa Medical College for 3 years in rotation in all the departments especially in paediatrics and gynaecology. That experience helped in my practice but more importantly I then learnt that the diagnosis is the same in both streams of medicine and that allopathic medicine varies only in treatment from homeopathy.

Today homeopathy has been a great help especially to women and children. I see more women and children in my clinic. Women have a lot of 'unaddressed' health concerns, related to overwork, stress and depression. As they have invariably the major burden of bringing up children, house hold chores, and work outside the home. Women today have lot of responsibilities to face the challenges of life on their own. Most often without help from their husbands. Added to this is the fact that today's generation have much more stress and grow with tremendous anxiety and problems. These problems aggravate and trigger psychological and mental disorders, which need to be cured and taken care of without pain or side effects.

In the clinics the common complaints of the women is handling menopause and girls is puberty. Other complaints such as spondilytis, rheumatic disorders, osteo-arthritis, cruelty, psychic problems. Some complaints are due to stress and here homeopathy works excellently without giving any side effects. Homeopathy does not make use of hormones or tranquilizers or antibiotics. Patients don't get any stomach upsets or acidity and everybody can digest it well. As powerful drugs are never administered to the patient however it is selected according to her constitution. Homeopathy is sometimes a slow acting but a sure cure medication for the problem.

Coming to children, the child's constitution is tender and when homeopathic drugs are administered the response is quicker. The problem with children is generally common colds, skin disease, allergic problems, and nutritional disorders. If these are rectified at an earlier stage the child is sure to grow strong and healthy physically and mentally. They develop their immunity and most often they learn to discipline themselves with food habits which is otherwise a big problem for mothers to handle. As medicines are sweet in taste all the children take it easily and children remind the mother if she forgets to give the dosage.

The child learns to be regular with medication and certainly the child develops attitudes to be systematic in his life. This medication is continuous but tapered and therefore the patient has to be regularly guided and reassured. A very supportive and a constant reassurance from the part of the practitioner is of utmost importance.

Children grow with a positive attitude towards life and do not develop negative feelings as they can cope with life's stormy days with great ease. They learn to recognise their own body system and its functioning and will immediately report any weakness experienced so that they can visit the doctor immediately. Attendance in schools in generally regular and they do not miss out on any assignments on a regular basis. I see in my clinic a number of times a mother brings one child to the clinic, then on her second visit, she brings the second child and then on the third visit she becomes a patient because she prefers to be treated with homeopathy as it suits them well.

No doubt, Homeopathy, had not dug a strong foundation in the 60s. However, today, women are very keen on their choice of medication. Education has played an important role in the study of science. The knowledge of side/after effects of several allopathic medicines has made people prefer this harmless medication. Homeopathy has proved that it is a medication with no side effects and definitely it is the reason why educated mother will always find it their choice. It has been able to provide long-term cure and relief diseases like Athritis, Rheumatic disorders, Asthma, liver diseases, skin disorders and if treated at the initial stage and proper guidance by experienced homeopaths has proved for itself.

The system treats the patient as a whole and tries to make a comprehensive assessment of the body's reaction to the pathogenic factors. It is therefore very important that the patient's case history should be carefully noted down. Primary emphasis is laid on therapeutics and takes a holistic approach towards the sick individual and treats his disturbances on the physical, emotional and mental levels at the same time.

It aims at bringing back the best equilibrium of the sick individual on all three levels by stimulating and strengthening his body's defence mechanism. Homeopathy is concerned with the persons temperament, dreams, likes, dislikes, food preferences, tastes etc.

The classical approach to the problem being individualistic, the practitioner has to have a detailed and long interviews to find out specific characteristics of the defence mechanism of each sick person even though a group may be suffering of the same disease. Homeopathy allows patients to ventilate and talk that often a patient may feel better without medicines. Coping with the high cost of living, homeopathy suits perfectly any individual's pocket being low cost and a non-toxic drug with its benefits to human health being highly commendable.

Over the years, the Government of India has extended a broad policy support to the study of Homeopathy and provided manpower and financial resources. It is therefore of vital importance that this system of medicine should be given due recognition. The public should definitely awaken to re- enforce, to make an organised attempt to integrate the genius of this system in a meaningful manner in the health care activities. Health Centres should have outlets for Homeopathic practitioners as well. The cost of such centres will be marginal and will not be of any financial burden to the Government. The choice of the system of medicine lies entirely on the individual. As the constitution supports its citizens freedom. Today the Goan population is increasing due to the influx of its residents and tourists. Pollutants have caused a number of allergic diseases. I see little children being affected tremendously with ailments where in mothers rush sometimes with all the members of the family suffering of the same ailment.

Today in my private clinic, I am getting more referral patients from paediatrician and skin specialists because they have seen the results on an average 30/40 patients a day. Therefore establishing the fact that the demand for homeopathy does exist. In the government clinic patients were mostly poor patients but in private practice the clients are from all walks of life. The working class who could not attend day clinics come to the private clinic after work.

I conclude this paper with a proposal.

- To recognise the value of the science.
- As it serves the women population. Mothers who bring their children to the clinics often get their own problems addressed to as well.
- Medicines in allopathy are often too strong, and sometimes have side effects. They are particularly hard for children to digest.
- Some illness do get cured with allopathy.
- Homeopathy delves in detail into the individual as a person and not just as a patient with certain symptoms. Other medical practices don't really concern themselves

with a persons temperament, dreams, likes, dislikes, food preferences etc.

- The homeopathy clinics allow patients to ventilate and talk that often a patient may feel better even without medicines.
- History taking done the way it is in homeopathic practice is important for diagnosis and treatment and also serves as a way of counselling as mentioned above. This also allows for referral of the patient for professional help.
- In homeopathy there is preventive medicine just like vaccinations etc. but for other illnesses like asthma etc.
- Finally and most importantly, the investment required by homeopathy, including the medicines is very little while it can serve a large population. The approximate investment to give a rough picture is about Rs. 20,000 (not including salaries) for one years medicines. It will be cheaper if the tender is larger. This figure will service a population of thousands. Besides the staff required for a homeopathic clinic is only one doctor, one compounder and a peon.
- To strengthen the scope of Homeopathy care in Goa. I feel more Homeopathic clinics should be opened in all urban and primary centres under a separate Directorate of Homeopathy and Indian Systems of Medicine like other states.
- In villages and remote places where the system of medicine is still not known field workers from the health centres should be trained to propagate these science and mobile clinics to be started for those patients who cannot attend the OPD regularly transport difficulties.

# INDEX